CONTENTS

I0758215

GOOD FOOD
GOOD HEALTH

THE SECRET OF GOOD HEALTH

Dedication

To the memory of my father

Joel Matthew

who taught me the

Principles of life.

ABOUT THIS BOOK

Good Food Good Health, best-selling author and leading expert Solomon O. Matthew shares his formula for lifelong vitality. This book will arm you with the information that will help you to make the right choices about your food in order for you to stay alive and well.

this book clearly explains the intricacies of each problem and offers useful tips on how to truly make a difference through diet. The recipes provided for each imbalance are easy to follow and are accompanied by detailed nutritional information. The information throughout the book, including the chapter on Blood type diet, is designed for clients who wish to optimize their health, whether or not they are currently facing health problems with food.

With focus on a personalized approach to helping people through diet, this book is an invaluable resource for nutritionists, health professionals and their clients.

ACKNOWLEDGEMENTS

I appreciate the support and co-operation of my peaceful and loving family that I enjoy from time to time especially during the period of producing this work.

Everyone listed here has made significant contributions to the writing of this book.They are listed in no particular order. Many thanks to Mr Olawale Lateef, Mr Tosin babs, Pst Awolowo Segun, Fajana Taiwo, Joshua Oladele, Ezekiel Oladipo, Tobe Adesanya, Oyebade Dada, Shittu Keji, Ololade Lateef, Olabode Matthew, Bashir Ramon, Adeyemo Ifeoluwa, Makinde Afeez, Deanne Edwards and Steve Shaw.

CHAPTER ONE

INTRODUCTION

FOOD has been a fundamental piece of our reality. Through the centuries we have gained riches of data about the utilization of food to guarantee development of children, youth and old, to maintain great wellbeing through life, and to address exceptional issues of pregnancy and lactation and to utilize it to recuperate from ailment. At the point when you concentrate on food composition you will know the nourishing commitment of food varieties. You may have been informed that specific food sources are vital for keeping up with great wellbeing, while others are destructive. As you concentrate on the study of Foods and Nutrition, you should inspect the thoughts you have about food varieties cautiously and acknowledge or dismiss these in the knowledge of the information you will obtain.

Anything that you learn in this space ought to be utilized and applied in your own life.

A large part of our food legacy is experimentally valuable and should be retained; maybe a few viewpoints ought to be adjusted in the perspective on the progressions in our way of life.

Food is a significant subject of discussions, articles in papers and magazines, as likewise of commercials. A portion of this data might be right, however an enormous piece of it may not be. As you learn this subject, you will be able to spread the knowledge gained to those around you, so that they discard false ideas about food, which interfere with their food selection and affect their health. Food, nutrition and health are intimately connected aspects of our life. Let us start our study by defining these and related terms

Definitions

Food is that which nourishes the body. Food may likewise be characterized as anything eaten or drunk, which addresses the issues for energy, building, regulation and protection of the body. To put it plainly, food is the natural substance from which our bodies are made. Intake of the right sorts and measures of food can guarantee great nourishment and wellbeing, which might be clear in our appearance, effectiveness and emotional well-being.

Nourishment has been characterized as food at work in the body. Nutrition incorporates all that occurs to food from the time it is eaten until it is utilized for different capabilities in the body. Nutrition is parts of food that are required by the body in sufficient sums to develop healthy life. Nutrition incorporates water, proteins, fats, carbohydrates, minerals and vitamins. There are a few supplements in every one of the groups: proteins, fats, carbohydrates, minerals and vitamins; consequently, the plural type of these words has been utilized. Along these lines there are more than 40 fundamental supplements provided by food which are used to produce literally thousands of substances necessary for life and physical fitness.

The study of the science of nutrition deals with what nutrients we need, how much we need, why we want these and where we can get them. Nutrition is the aftereffect of the sorts of food sources provided to the body and how the body utilizes the food provided.

Adequate nutrition are expressions used to indicate that the supply of the essential nutrients is correct in amount and proportion. It likewise implies that the use of such Nutrition in the body is to such an extent that the most significant level of physical and emotional wellness is kept up with all through the life-cycle.

Nutritional status is the condition of our body because of the food varieties ate and their utilization by the body. Nourishing status can be great, fair or poor.

The qualities of good nourishing status are a ready, natured personality, a well created body, with normal weight for height, well developed and firm muscles, healthy skin, and reddish pink color of eyelids and membranes of mouth, good layer of subcutaneous fat, clear eyes, smooth and glossy hair, good appetite and excellent general health. General good health is evident by stamina for work, regular meal times, sound regular sleep, normal elimination and resistance to disease.

Poor nutritional status is evidenced by a listless, apathetic or irritable personality, undersized poorly developed body, strange body weight (too flimsy or fat and heavy body), muscles little and overweight, pale or pallid skin, too little or an excess of subcutaneous fat, dull or blushed eyes, lusterless and harsh hair, unfortunate craving, absence of life and perseverance for work and defenselessness to contaminations. Poor nourishing status might be the result of poor food selection, irregularity in schedule of meals, work, sleep and elimination.
The WHO (World Health Organization) has characterized health as the 'state of complete physical, mental and social well-being and not merely the absence of disease or infirmity'.

Malnutrition means an unfortunate kind of nutrition leading to chronic sickness. It results from a need, overabundance or awkwardness of supplements in the eating routine. It incorporates under nutrition and over nutrition. Under nutrition is a state of an insufficient supply of essential nutrients while Over nutrition refers to an excessive intake of one or more nutrients, which creates a stress in the bodily function.

Diet refers to anything you eat and drink every day. Thus, it includes the normal diet you consume and the diet people consume in groups (hostel diet). Diet may likewise be adjusted and utilized for sick people as a feature of their treatment.

Nutritional care is the use of nutritional knowledge in planning meals and the preparation of these meals in an acceptable and attractive manner to feed people. It includes evaluation of the exiting meal patterns and working on these in a satisfactory way. While the dietary arrangement might be general for a gathering, the genuine execution is individualized to suit the individual's requirements and foundation.

Hence one needs to utilize a ton of resourcefulness to prevail with regards to making nourishing consideration successful in reasonable terms.

Health the word health refers to the state of the body, good health not only implies freedom from disease, but physical, mental and emotional fitness as well.

Function of Food

Physiological function of food. The principal capability of the body is to give energy. The body needs energy to support the compulsory cycle's fundamental for duration of life, to carry out professional, household and recreational activities, to convert food ingested into usable nutrients in the body, to develop and to keep warm. The energy required is provided by the oxidation of the food consumed.

The food varieties we eat become a part of us. In this manner one of the main elements of food is building the body. An infant weighing 2.7-3.2 kg can develop to its expected grown-up size of 50-60 kg in the event that the right sorts and measures of food are eaten from birth to adulthood. The food eaten every day assists with keeping up with the structure of the adult body, and to replace broken down cells of the body.

The third function of food is to control activities of the body. It includes guideline of such varied activities as:
• Beating of the heart
• Upkeep of the internal heat level
• Muscle compression
• Control of water balance
•Clotting of blood
• Expulsion of side-effects from the body
The fourth function of food is to work on our body's protection

from sickness.

The Social Functions of Food. Food has forever been a focal part of our social existence. It has been a part of our community, social, cultural and religious life. Food has been utilized as a statement of affection, friendship and social acceptance. It is additionally utilized as an image of joy at specific occasions throughout everyday life.

As food is a necessary part of our social existence, this capability is significant in day-to-day existence.

Refreshments served at get-togethers or meetings create a relaxed atmosphere. The menu for such get-together ought to unite individuals, instead of separation them. This fundamental angle ought to be thought about in arranging menus for such events.

The Psychological Functions of Food. As well as fulfilling physical and social necessities, food should fulfill specific feelings. This includes a sense of security, love and attention. Thus, familiar foods make us feel secure. Anticipating needs and fulfilling these are expressions of love and attention. These sentiments are the basis of the normal attachment to the mother's cooking.

Sharing of food is a token of companionship and acknowledgment. In a cordial social gathering we try unfamiliar foods and thus enlarge our food experiences. It should be noticed that even a healthfully adjusted dinner may not be fulfilling to the individual, if the foods included are unfamiliar or distasteful to him/her.

Elements of Nutrients

The food sources which we utilize everyday include rice, wheat, vegetables, natural products, milk, eggs, fish, meat, sugar, margarine, oils, and so on. These various food varieties are comprised of various substance parts called nutrients. These are characterized by their chemical composition.

Every nutrient class has its own capability; however, the different nutrients should act as one for compelling activity. The nutrients found in food sources are — carbohydrates, fats, minerals, vitamins and water.

Fiber is likewise a fundamental part of our eating routine. The elements of nutrients are given below.

Carbohydrates:	Starch found in cereals and sugar in sugarcane and natural products are instances of carbohydrates in food varieties. The main capability of carbohydrates is to give energy required by our body.

Those not utilized quickly for this object are put away as glycogen or changed over completely to fat and put away, to be assembled for energy supply when required.

Fats: Oils found in seeds, margarine from milk, and fat from meat, are examples of fats found in food varieties. Fats are concentrated sources of energy, transporters of fat-soluble vitamins and a source of fundamental fatty acids. In the event that abundance fats are taken in the eating routine, these are put away as fat stores in the body.

Proteins: Casein from milk, albumin in egg, globulins in vegetables and gluten in wheat, are models of proteins happening in food sources. The primary capability of protein is the building of new tissues and maintaining and repair of those already built. Synthesis of regulatory and protective substances such as enzymes, hormones and antibodies are also a function of food proteins. About 10 per cent of the total energy is supplied by proteins in the diet. Protein, when taken in excess of the body's need, is converted to carbohydrates and fats and is stored in the body.

Minerals: The minerals calcium, phosphorus, iron, iodine, sodium, potassium and others are tracked down in different food varieties in blend with natural and inorganic mixtures. Minerals are vital for body-building, for building of bones, teeth and structural parts of soft tissues. They likewise assume a part in guideline of cycles in the body, e.g., muscle contraction, clotting of blood, nerve improvements, and so on.

Vitamins: Fat- soluble vitamins A, D, E and K and furthermore water- soluble vitamins C and B group are found in food varieties. These are required for development, normal function of the body and normal body processes.

Water: We get water in food sources we eat and a significant part from the water we drink in that capacity and as refreshments. Water is a fundamental part of our body construction and it represents around 60% of our body weight. Water is fundamental for the utilization of food material in the body and furthermore for disposal of food waste. It is a regulator of body processes such as maintenance of body temperature.

All individuals need similar supplements for a similar body capability. The main variety is in the measures of every supplement expected by age, size, movement, and so forth. For instance, all people need energy for work, however a man, who carries loads might require more energy than, a man who works in an office at a desk job.

CHAPTER TWO

BLOOD CODE: THE BLUEPRINT OF BLOOD TYPE

BLOOD IS A power of nature, the ELAN VITAL that has supported us since time immemorial. A solitary drop of blood, too little to even consider seeing with the naked eye, contains the whole hereditary code of an individual. The DNA blueprint is intact and replicated within us endlessly- through our blood.

Our blood likewise contains an age of hereditary memory-- pieces and bits of explicit programming, passed on from our precursors in codes we are as yet endeavoring to grasp. One such code rests inside our blood type. Maybe it is the main code we can translate in our endeavor to unwind the secrets of blood and its vital role in our existence.

To the naked eye, blood is a homogenous red fluid. Yet, under the microscope blood shows itself to be made out of a wide range of components. The plentiful red platelets contain an exceptional kind of iron that our bodies use to convey oxygen and make the blood's characteristic rust color. White blood cells, far less numerous than red, cruise our bloodstreams like ever-vigilant troops, protecting us against infection. This intricate, living liquid additionally contains proteins that convey supplements to the tissues, platelets that assist it with thickening and plasma that contains the guardians of our immune system.

-The Importance of Blood

Type. You may be unaware of your own blood type unless you've donated blood or needed a transfusion. Most people think of blood type as an inert factor, something that only comes into play when there is a hospital emergency. But now that you have heard the dramatic story of the evolution of blood type, you are beginning to understand that blood type has always been the driving force behind human survival, changing and adapting to new conditions, environments and foods supplies.

Why is our blood type so powerful? What is the essential role it plays in our survival--not just thousands of years ago, but today?

Your blood type is the key to your body's entire immune system. It controls the influence of viruses, bacteria, infections, chemicals, stress and the entire assortment of invaders and conditions that might compromise your immune system.

The word 'immune' comes from the Latin IMMUNIS, which denoted a city in the Roman Empire that was not required to pay taxes. (If only your blood type could give you that kind of immunity!) The immune system works to define 'self' and destroy 'non self. This is a critical function, for without it your immune system could attack your own tissues by mistake or allow a dangerous organism access to vital areas of your body. In spite of all its complexity, the immune system boils down to two basic functions: recognizing 'us' and killing 'them'. In this respect your body is like a large invitation-only party. If the prospective guest supplies the correct invitation, the security guards allow him to enter and enjoy himself. If an invitation is lacking or forged, the guest is forcefully removed.

-Enter the Blood Type.

Nature has enriched our immune systems with exceptionally modern techniques to decide whether a substance in the body is unfamiliar or not. One technique includes substance markers called ANTIGENS which are tracked down on our bodies. Each living thing, from the least difficult infection to people themselves, has extraordinary antigens that structure a piece of their chemicals fingerprint. Perhaps of the most remarkable antigen in the human body is the one that decides your blood classification. The different blood type antigens are delicate to such an extent that when they are working successfully, they are the resistant framework's most prominent security framework. At the point when your immune system sizes up a suspicious character (for example an unfamiliar antigen from bacteria) one of the primary things it searches for is your blood classification antigen to tell it whether the interloper is companion or enemy. Each blood classification has an alternate antigen with its own exceptional compound design. Your blood classification is named for [sic] the blood classification antigen you have on your red cells.

IF YOU ARE: ANTIGEN(S) ON YOUR CELLS
Blood Type A: A.
Blood Type B: B.
Blood Type AB: A and B.
Blood Type O: no antigens.

Visualize the chemical structure of blood types as antennae of sorts, projecting outwards from the surface of our cells into deep space. These antennae are made from long chains of a repeating sugar called fucose, which by itself forms the simplest of the blood types, the O antigen of Blood Type O. The early discoveries of blood type called it 'O' as a way to make us think of 'zero' or 'no real antigen'. This antenna also serves as the base for the other Blood Types, A, B and AB.

__ Blood Type A is formed when the O antigen, or fucose, plus another sugar called N-acetyl-galactosamine, is added. So, fucose plus N-acetyl-galactosamine equals Blood Type A.

__ Blood Type B is also based on the O antigen, or fucose, but has a different sugar, named D-galactosamine, added on. So, fucose plus D-galactosamine equals Blood Type B.

__ Blood Type AB is based on the O antigen, fucose, plus the two sugars, Nicety-galactosamine and D-galactosamine. So, fucose plus N-acetyl-galactosamine plus D-galactosamine equals Blood Type AB.

At this point you may be wondering about other blood type identifiers, like positive and negative, or secretor/non-secretor. Usually, when people state their blood types they say, 'I'm A positive' or, 'I'm O negative'. These variations, or sub-groups, within blood types play relatively insignificant roles. More than 90 per cent of all the factors associated with your blood type are related to your primary type--O, A, B, or AB. (See Appendix E for details on the meaning of the subgroups.) We will concentrate on your blood type itself.

-Antigens Create Antibodies (Immune System Smart Bombs).

At the point when your blood classification antigen detects that an unfamiliar antigen has entered the system, the primary thing it does is make antibodies to that antigen. These antibodies, specific synthetic substances fabricated by the cells of the insusceptible system, are intended to append to and label the unfamiliar antigen for destruction.

Antibodies are what might be compared to the military's smart bomb. The cells of our immune system make endless assortments of antibodies, and each is explicitly intended to recognize and join to one specific unfamiliar antigen. A continual battle wages between the immune system and intruders who try to change or mutate their antigens into some new form that the body will not recognize. The immune system answers this test with a steadily expanding stock of antibodies.

At the point when an immunizer experiences the antigen of a microbial intruder, a response called agglutination (gluing) happens. The antibody joins itself to the viral antigen and makes it extremely tacky. At the point when cells, infections, parasites and bacteria are agglutinated, they remain together and bunch up, which makes the occupation of their removal all the more straightforward. As microorganisms should depend on their dangerous powers of avoidance, this is an extremely strong protection component. It is fairly similar to cuffing lawbreakers together; they become definitely less hazardous than when they are permitted to move around freely. Sweeping the system of odd cells, viruses, parasites and bacteria, the antibodies herd the undesirables together for easy identification and disposal.

The system of blood type antigens and antibodies has other ramifications besides detecting microbial and other invaders. Nearly a century ago, Dr. Karl Landsteiner, a brilliant Austrian physician and scientist, also found that blood types produced antibodies to other blood types. His revolutionary discovery explained why some people could exchange blood, while others could not. Until Dr. Landsteiner's time, blood transfusions were a hit and miss affair. Sometimes they 'took', and sometimes they didn't and nobody knew why. Thanks to Dr. Landsteiner, we now know which blood types are recognized as friend by other blood types, and which are recognized as foe. Dr. Landsteiner learned that:

__ Blood Type A carried anti-B antibodies. Type B would be rejected by Type A.

__ Blood Type B carried anti-A antibodies. Type A would be rejected by Type B.

_Thus, Type A and Type B could not exchange blood. _

__ Blood Type AB carried no antibodies. The universal receiver, it would accept any other blood type! But, because it carried both A and B antigens, it would be rejected by all other blood types.

Thus, Type AB could receive blood from everyone, but could give blood to no one (except another Type AB, of course).

__ Blood Type O carried anti-A and anti-B antibodies. Type A, Type B and Type AB would be rejected.

Thus, Type O could not receive blood from anyone but another Type O. But, free of A-like and B-like antigens, Type O could give blood to everyone else. Type O is the universal donor!

IF YOU ARE:	YOU CARRY ANTIBODIES AGAINST.
Blood Type A:	Blood Type B.
Blood Type B:	Blood Type A.
Blood Type AB:	No antibodies.
Blood Type O:	Blood Type A and B.

The 'anti-other-blood-type' antibodies are the strongest antibodies in our immune system, and their ability to clump (agglutinate) the blood cells of an opposing blood type is so powerful that it can be immediately observed on a glass slide with the unaided eye. Most of our other antibodies require some sort of stimulation (such as a vaccination or an infection) for their production. The blood type antibodies are different: they are produced automatically, often appearing at birth and reaching almost adult levels by four months of age.

But there is much more to the agglutination story. It was also found that many foods agglutinate the cells of certain blood types (in a way similar to rejection) but not others, meaning that a food which may be harmful to the cells of one blood type may be beneficial to the cells of another. Not surprisingly, many of the antigens in these foods had A-like or B-like characteristics. This discovery provided the scientific link between blood type and diet. Remarkably, however, its revolutionary implications would lie dormant, gathering dust for most of this century--until a handful of scientists, doctors and nutritionists began to explore the connection.

Lectins: The Diet Connection.

A chemical reaction occurs between your blood and the foods that you eat. This reaction is part of your genetic inheritance. It is amazing but true that today, in the late twentieth century, your immune and digestive systems still maintain a favoritism for foods that your blood type ancestors ate.

We know this because of a factor called lectins. Lectins, abundant and diverse proteins found in foods, have agglutinating properties that affect your blood. Lectins are a powerful way for organisms to attach themselves to other organisms in nature. Lots of germs, and even our own immune systems, used this super-glue to their benefit. For example, cells in our liver's bile ducts have lectins on their surfaces to help them snatch up bacteria and parasites. Bacteria and other microbes have lectins on their surfaces, as well, which work rather like suction cups, so they can attach to the slippery mucosal linings of the body. Often, the lectins used by viruses or bacteria can be blood type specific, making them a stickier pest for a person of that blood type.

So, too, with the lectins in food. When you eat a food containing protein lectins that are incompatible with your blood type antigen, the lectins target an organ or bodily system (kidney, liver, brain, stomach, etc.) and begin to agglutinate blood cells in that area.

Many food lectins have characteristics that are close enough to a certain blood type antigen to make it an 'enemy' to another. For example, milk has B-like qualities; if a person with Type A blood drinks it, their system will immediately start the agglutination process in order to reject it.

Here's an example of how a lectin agglutinates in the body. Let's say a Type A person drinks a glass of milk. The milk is digested in the stomach through the process of acid hydrolysis. However, the lectin protein is resistant to acid hydrolysis. It doesn't get digested, but stays intact. It may interact directly with the lining of the stomach or intestinal tract, or it may get absorbed into our bloodstream along with the digested nutrients. Different lectins target different organs and body systems.

Once the intact lectin protein settles somewhere in your body, it literally has a magnetic effect on the cells in that region. It clumps the cells together and they are targeted for destruction, as if they, too, were foreign invaders. This clumping can cause irritable bowel syndrome in the intestines, cirrhosis of the liver, or block the flow of blood through the kidneys--to name just a few of the effects.

Lectins: A Dangerous Glue.

You may remember the bizarre assassination of Gyorgi Markov in 1978 on a London Street. Markov was killed by an unknown Soviet KGB agent while waiting for a bus. Initially, the autopsy could not pinpoint how it was done. After a thorough search, however, a tiny gold bead was found embedded in Markov's leg. The bead was found to be permeated with a chemical called ricin, which is a toxic lectin extracted from castor beans. Ricin is so potent an agglutinin that even an infinitesimally small amount can cause death by swiftly converting the body's red blood cells into large clots which block the arteries. Ricin kills instantaneously.

Fortunately, most lectins found in the diet are not quite so life-threatening, although they can cause a variety of other problems, especially if they are specific to a particular blood type. For the most part our immune systems protect us from lectins. Ninety-five per cent of the lectins we absorb from our typical diets are sloughed off by the body. But at least 5 per cent of the lectins we eat are filtered into the blood stream, where they react with and destroy red and white blood cells. The actions of lectins in the digestive tract can be even more powerful. There, they often create a violent inflammation of the sensitive mucus of the intestines, and this agglutinative action may mimic food allergies. Even a minute quantity of a lectin is capable of agglutinating a huge number of cells if the particular blood type is reactive.

This is not to say that you should suddenly become fearful of every food you eat. After all, lectins are widely abundant in pulses seafood, grains and vegetables. It's hard to bypass them. The key is to avoid the lectins that agglutinate your particular cells-determined by blood type. For example, gluten, the most common lectin found in wheat and other grains, binds to the lining of the small intestine, causing substantial inflammation and painful irritation in some blood types--especially Type O.

Lectins vary widely according to their source. For example, the lectin found in wheat has a different shape and attaches to a different combination of sugars than the lectin found in soya, making each of these foods dangerous for some blood types, but beneficial for others.

Nervous tissue as a rule is very sensitive to the agglutinating effect of food lectins. This may explain why some researchers feel that allergy-avoidance diets may be of benefit in treating certain types of nervous disorders, such as hyperactivity, Russian researchers have noted that the brains of schizophrenics are more sensitive to the attachment of certain common food lectins.

Injections of lentil lectin into the knee-joint cavities of non-sensitized rabbits resulted in the development of arthritis that was indistinguishable from rheumatoid arthritis. Many people with arthritis feel that avoiding the so-called 'nightshade' vegetables, such as tomatoes, auberges and white potatoes, seems to help their arthritis. That's not surprising, since most nightshades are very high in lectins.

Food lectins can also interact with the surface receptors of the body's white cells, programming them to multiply rapidly. These lectins are called mitogens because they cause the white cells to enter mitosis, the process of cell reproduction. They do not clump blood by gluing cells together; they merely attach themselves to things, like fleas on a dog. Occasionally an emergency room doctor will be faced with a very ill but otherwise apparently normal child who has an extraordinarily high white blood cell count. Although pediatric leukemia is usually the first thing to come to mind, the astute doctor will ask the parent, 'Was your child playing in the garden?' If the answer is yes, 'Was he eating any weeds or putting plants in his mouth?' It may turn out that the child was eating the leaves or shoots of the North American pokeweed plant, which contains a lectin with the potent ability to stimulate white cell production.

CHAPTER THREE

FOUR THINGS YOU SHOULO KNOW ABOUT FOOD

The desire of everyone is to live as many years as possible. However, life expectancy on earth has been decreasing with increasing in age and technology. Research has shown that most of the world life threatening diseases like cancer, heart diseases etc. have their blood sugar levels by our and lifestyles have been implicated in most diseases. Various studies in the past have suggested that blood group is one of the main genetic factors that affect health and well-being to a larger extent. There are essentially four main types of blood groups that include A, B, O and AB. It is imperative to follow your diet according to the blood type as people with different blood groups digest lectins in a different way. The blood group tends to determine how the body deals with different nutrients. Therefore, following a 'blood type diet' is important. Blood type diet is basically based on eating specific foods in order to facilitate better digestion, increase energy levels and prevent certain diseases and ailments. If we look at some of the basic medical factors that affect an individual's weight and fitness levels, be it a person's ideal body weight, diet, food allergies, sleep pattern and general medical history, the Blood type diet does not cater to any of these factors. It removes all the processed foods and most of the simple carbohydrates from the diet.

The tour things you should know about food that will help you to be free from food induced diseases are as follows:

1. Two types of food

2. Three forms of food

3. The right way to eat

4. Healthy food preparations.

All these are explained in details in this book. Once you have the knowledge of these four things, try as much as possible to put the knowledge to use. A great philosopher, Napoleon Hill once said "it is not more education, it is not more knowledge, it is not more fact that we need to have but a better use of what we already have is what we need to have.' The law of cause and effect says there is a specific effect for every cause. For every action there is a reaction. The law implies here that neither health nor sickness is accident. The law is no respecter of people, places or situations one must just do the needful to be in health and if one fails to do the needful, sickness is inevitable. The choice is ours to make: It is not what we wish for; we just must do what we need to do. To be able to do this, it requires determination and discipline.

NATURAL CHOICE 1ST CHOICE	MODERATELY PROCESSED 2ND CHOICE	HIGHLY PROCESSED LIMIT	SHOPPING TIP
CORN ON THE COB	POP CORN	CORNFLAKES	Buy popcorn t- and eat in moderatio n and limit the intake of cornflakes.
PEACH	CANNED PEACHES IN 100% JUICE	CANNED PEACHES IN HEAVY SYRUP	Fruit canned is heavy syrup has more sugar and calories then fresh
FRESH FOODS	REFRIGERATED FOOD	FROZEN FOODS	Frozen foods

			are dead food with no food enzyme. The fresher your food the better.
PINEAPPLE	CANED DICED PINEAPPLE	PINEAPPLE COCKTAIL CUP	Fresh pineapple is higher in vitamin C and A and beta-carotene then canned
YAM	POUNDED YAM	PONDO YAM	Poundo yam take much longer time to digest than pounded yam
ORANGE	100% ORANGE JUICE	ORANGE DRINK	Many fruit drinks contain high fructose corn syrup and little real juice
FRESH FIGS	FIG PRESERVERS	FIG SANDWICHES COOKIES	Packaged fruit cookies may contain refine sugar and preservation
PLAIN YOGURT	FLAVORED YOGURT	FLAVOVED YOGURT DRINK	Buy plain yogurt and flavor it at home with the honey or fresh fruits
CREAM	FAT-FREE HALF CREAM/HALF MILK	FLAVORED DAIRY CREAMER	Flavored dairy creamer is often made with coloring artificial flavor and corn syrup
BROWN RICE	WHITE RICE	FLAVORED INSTANT RICE	Brown rice unlike white hasn't had

			its fiber-rich layers of bran and germ removed
DRIED WHOLE WHEAT PASTA	DRIED WHITE PASTA	INSTANT NOODLES	Whole grain pasta is higher in antioxidants than white or instant noodles
WHOLE GRAIN BREAD	WHEAT BREAD	FORTIFIED WHITE BREAD	If a whole grain isn't the first ingredient, you missing out on nutrients
GARLIC	JARRED MINCED GARLIC	BOTTLED GARLIC MARINADE	Minced fresh garlic is cheaper and more flavor than jarred
SPINACH	BAGGED PRE-WASHED SPINACH	FRONZEN CREAMED SPINACH	Avoid frozen vegetable in sodium rice sauce, buy plain and add your own light sauce.
APPLE	APPLESAUCE	APPLE TOASTER PASRY	Applesauce is a healthy choice but it has fewer nutrient than whole apple
WHOLE SOYA BEANS	TOFU	FRONZEN VEGGIE BURGER	Frozen veggie burger is vegetarian friendly but are highly processed
PEANUTS	**NATURAL PEANUT BUTTER**	PROCESSED PEANUT BUTTER	Natural peanut butter should contain only peanuts and a dash of salt

GRASS FED BEEF	GRAIN FED BEEF	FRONEN BEEF PATTIES	Grass-fed beef is higher in nutrients and lower in fat than grain-feed beef
WHOLE TURKEY	DELI TURKEY	TURKEY MEAT BALLS	If you buy deli meat, ask brand free of filler and nitrates
CARROTS	BABY CARROTS	FROZEN HONEY GLAZED CARROTS	Baby carrots are healthy but more expensive than regular size loose carrots
HERITAGE HAM	DELI HAM	PACKAGED DELI BOLOGNA	Heritage varieties of pork are much less likely to contain hormones than factory meat
FRESH CHICKEN BREAST	DELI SLICED CHICKEN	CHICKEN NUGGETS	Chicken nuggets contain very little real chicken

THREE FORMS OF FOOD

The three forms of foods are:

1   Beneficial Foods

2   Neutral Foods

3   Detrimental Foods

1. Beneficial foods are foods that act like medicine in your body, food that is believed to be good for you because it does not contain artificial chemicals or much sugar or fat. They boast your immune system, help you to have normal weight, and help promote good sleep, give you energy and help you fight diseases.

2 Neutral foods are foods that you eat for eating sake. Neutral foods have neither an acidic nor alkaline effect on the body when consumed. They neither benefit you nor harm you. They are foods you eat for your stomach to just get filled up

3. Detrimental foods are foods that act like poison in your system; they are food that is not regarded as being conducive to maintaining good health, they are the triggers of diseases the accumulative effect of these foods over the years in the body results into different types of life-threatening diseases.

The Blood Group as the Determinant Factor

The determinant factor of the beneficial, neutral or detrimental is the blood group (O.A. B and AB) All (O) whether positive or negative reacts to the same foods, while AII (A) both positive and negative also reads to some foods and likewise all (B) and (AB) read to their own foods. These four common blood groups foods are explained in details in this book. These foods are in fifteen categories:

Dairy and eggs

Juices and Fluids

Vegetables

Meat and Poultry

Oils and Fats
Spices
Seafood

Fruits

Nuts and Seeds

Condiments

Grain and Pastas

Beverages

Bread and Muffins

Cereals

Beans and Legumes

CHAPTER FOUR

BLOOD GROUP A FOOD

AII group A flourish on vegetarian diets the inheritance of their more settled and less, war like farmers ancestors. This blood group should follow a meat-free diet, heavily based vegetables and fruits, legumes, beans and whole grains. The blood group A food also divides food in three forms: beneficial, neutral and detrimental. Beneficial foods are food that act like medicine, they help to fight diseases; the neutral foods neither benefit nor harm; while detrimental foods are foods that act like poison, they trigger diseases.

FOOD THAT PROMOTES WHEIGT LOSS FOR GROUP A

SOY FOODS aid efficient digestion, metabolize quickly

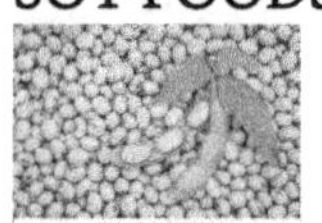

VEGETABLE OILS aid efficient digestion, prevent fluid retention

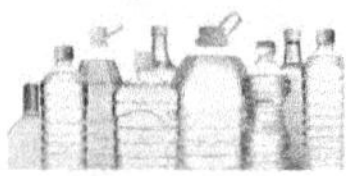

PINEAPLE increase calories utilization increases intestinal mobility

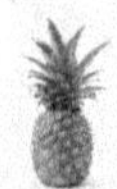

VEGETABLE aid efficient metabolism, increases intestinal mobility

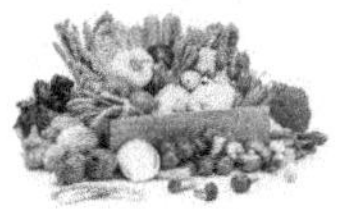

FOOD THAT PROMOTES WHEIGT GAIN FOR GROUP A

MEAT poorly digested, store as fat

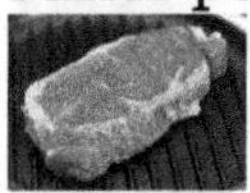

KIDNEY BEANS inactive digestive enzymes, slow metabolic rate

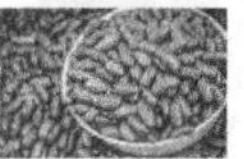

DAIRY FOOD inhabits nutrient metabolism

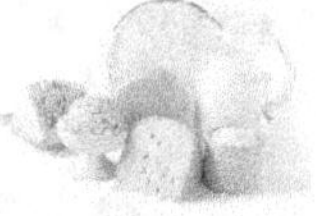

WHEAT IN OVER ABUNDANCE impair calorie utilization

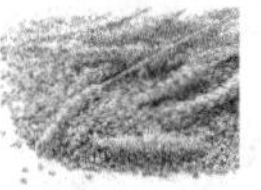

MEATS AND POULTRY

To receive the greatest benefits, Group As should eliminate all meats from their diet. It will take time for you to convert to a totally vegetarian diet. Be substituting fish for meat several times a week. When you eat meat, choose the leanest cuts you can find; poultry is preferred to red meat. Prepare meat by boiling or baking. Stay completely away from processed meat products, ham frankfurters, and cold cuts. They contain nitrites; promote stomach cancer in people with low levels of stomach acid - a group A trait.

Some natural meat for group A

Turkey   Chicken

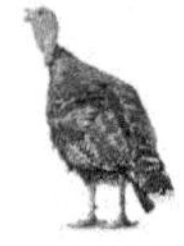 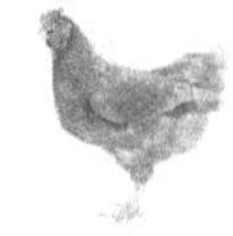

Some beneficial meat for group A

Group A should avoid meat.

Some detrimental meat for group A

Liver   Pork   Turtle

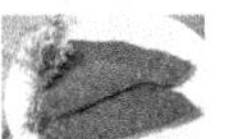 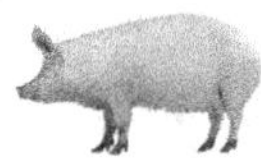 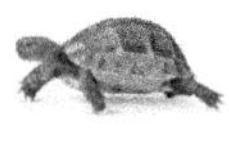

Beef   lamb

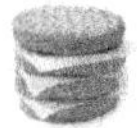 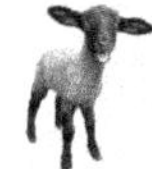

SEA FOODS

Group As can eat seafood in modest quantities three or four times a week, but should avoid white fish. They contain a lectin that can irritate the Group A digestive tract. If you are group A woman with history of breast cancer, consider introducing snails into your diet. Sea food should be baked or boiled to achieve its full nutritional value.

Some natural seafood for group A

Tilapia fish   Croaker fish

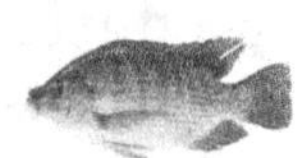 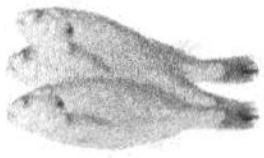

Some beneficial seafood for group A

Snail   Red snapper fish

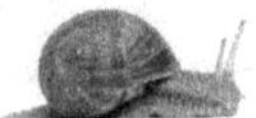 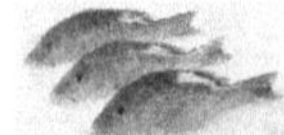

Some detrimental seafood for group A

Crab   White fish   Cat fish   Cray fish

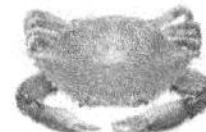 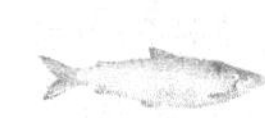 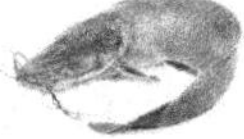 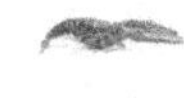

DAIRY AND EGG

Group A can tolerate small amounts of fermented dairy products, but should avoid anything made with whole milk, and limit egg consumption to occasional organically grown eggs. Group A normally produces more mucus than other blood groups. Too much mucus can be harmful, since various bacteria tend to live off it.

Some natural dairy and egg for group A

Butter   Yogurt   Duck egg

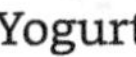
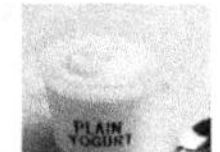 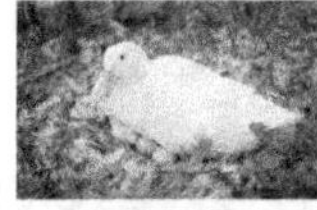
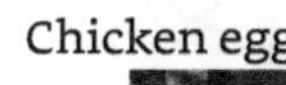

Quail egg   Goat milk   Chicken egg

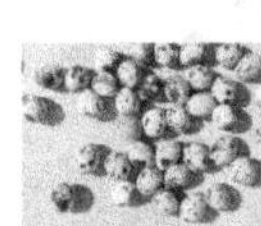 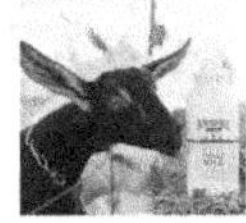 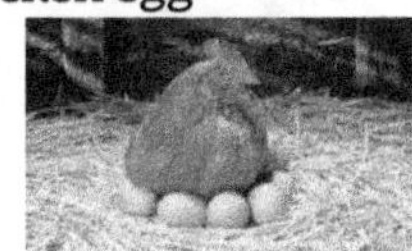

Some beneficial dairy and egg for group A

Type A individuals following the Blood Type diet are instructed to avoid all dairy products and eggs.

Some detrimental dairy and egg for group A

Cow milk
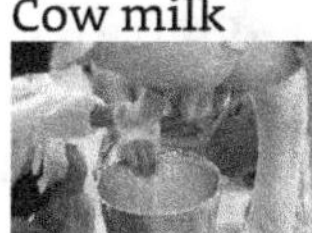

OILS AND FATS

Group As needs very little fat to function well, but a tablespoon of olive oil on salads or steamed vegetables every day will aid digestion and elimination. As a mono-saturated fat, olive oil also has a positive effect on your heart and may actually reduce cholesterol. The lectin in oils like corn oils cause problems in the group A digestive tract, Quite the opposite effect of the beneficial oil.

Some natural oil and fats for group A

Avocado oil   Cod liver oil   Almond oil

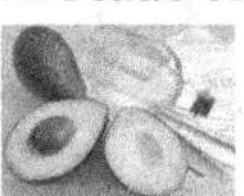  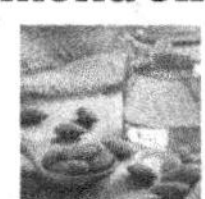

Some beneficial oil and fats for group A

Olive oil   Walnut oil

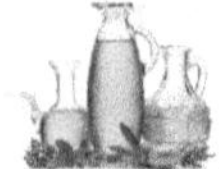 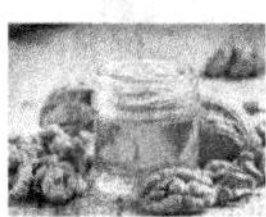

Some detrimental oil and fats for group A

Coconut oil   Corn oil

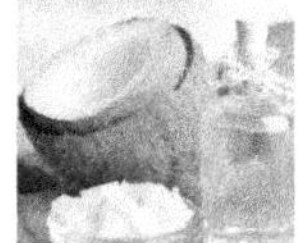 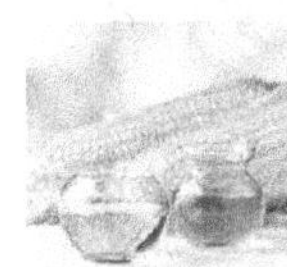

NUTS AND SEEDS

Many nuts and seeds, such as pumpkin and sunflower seeds, almonds, and walnuts, can provide positive supplementation for the Group A Diet. Since Group As eat very little animal protein, nuts and seeds supply an important protein component. Peanuts are the most beneficial. Eat them often because they contain a cancer-fighting lectin. Also eat the peanut skins (nut the shells). Pumpkin seeds are highly beneficial.

Some natural nuts and seeds for group A

Sesame seed

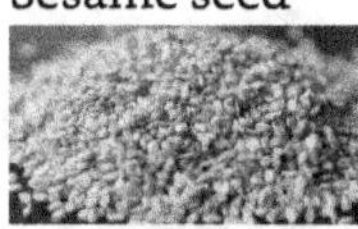

Almond

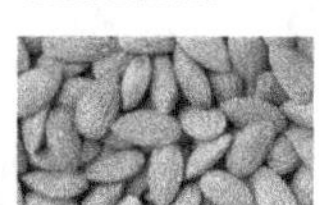

Sunflower seed

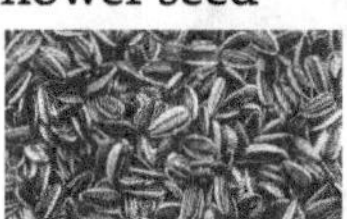

Some beneficial nuts and seeds for group A

Peanut

Pumpkin

Walnut

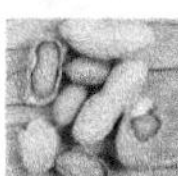

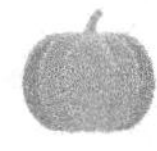

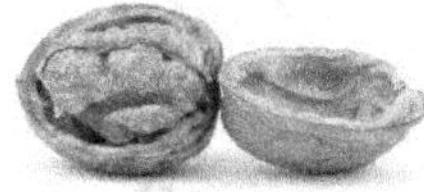

Some detrimental nuts and seeds for group A

Cashew nut

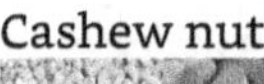
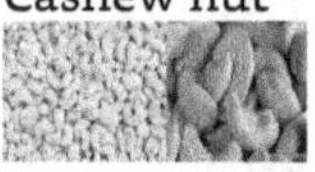

BEANS AND LEGUMES

Group A thrives on the vegetable proteins found in beans and legumes. Along with your friend the soybean, and all of its related products, many beans and legumes provide a nutritious source of protein. Be aware, however not all beans and legumes are good for you. Some, like the kidney, Lima and - navy contain a lectin that can cause a decrease in insulin production which is often a factor in obesity and diabetes.

Some natural beans and legumes beans for group A

Northern beans

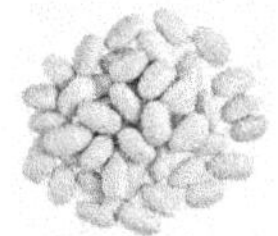

Some beneficial beans and legumes for group A

Pinto beans   adzuki beans

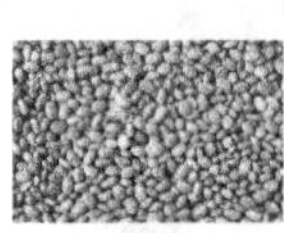 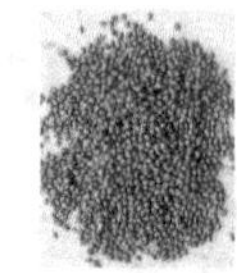

Some detrimental beans and legumes for group A

Kidney bean

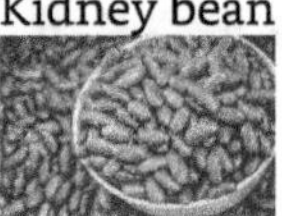

CEREAL

Group A generally does well on cereals and grains, and you can eat these foods once or more times a day. Select the more concentrated whole grains instead of instant and processed cereals. Introduce millet, soy wheat, cornmeal, and whole oats into your diet Group A with a pronounced mucus condition caused by asthma or frequent infections should limit wheat consumption as wheat causes mucus production.

Some natural cereals for group A

Cream of rice   Millet   Cornflakes   Tapioca

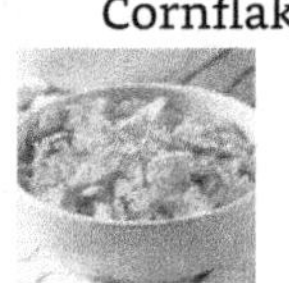 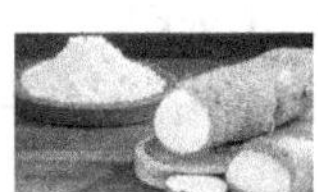

Some beneficial cereals for group A

Buck wheat   Oatmeal   Oat bran

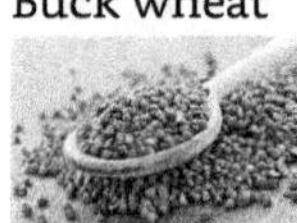 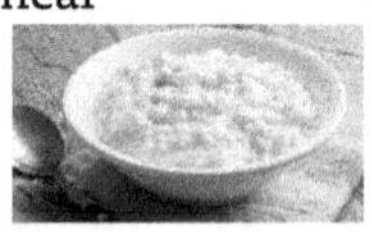 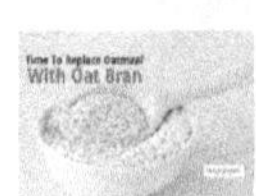

Some detrimental cereals for group A

Cream of wheat

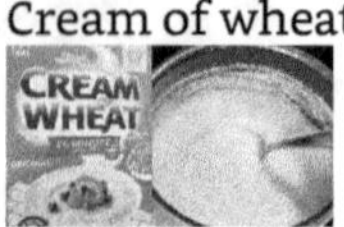

BREADS AND MUFFINS

The Group A guidelines for breads and muffins are similar to those of cereals and grains. They are generally favorable foods, but if you produce excessive mucus or are overweight, these conditions make whole wheat inadvisable. Soy and rice flour are good substitutes.

Some natural bread for group A

Brown rice bread

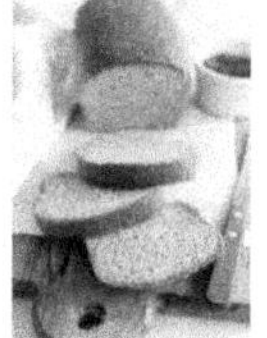

Some beneficial bread for group A

Essene

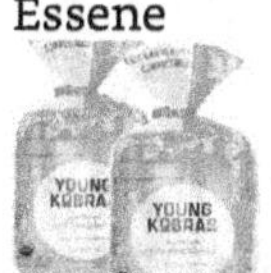

Some detrimental bread for group A

Whole wheat bread

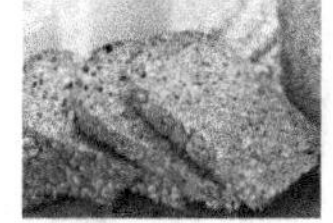

GRAINS AND PASTA

Group A has many choices in grains and pastas. These foods are excellent sources of vegetable protein. They can provide many of the nutrients that the group A is no longer receiving from animal protein, Stay away from processed products such as frozen meals, prepared noodles with sauces. Etc.,

Some natural grains and pastas for group A

Rice flour   Durum wheat flour

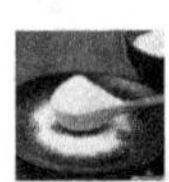 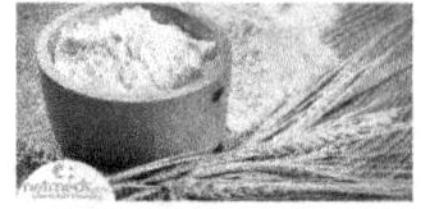

Some beneficial grains and pastas for group A

Saba noodle   Oat flour   Buck wheat

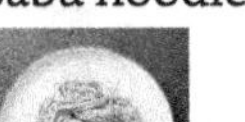 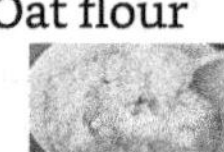 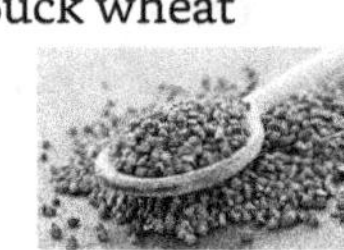

Some detrimental grains and pastas for group A

Whole wheat flour

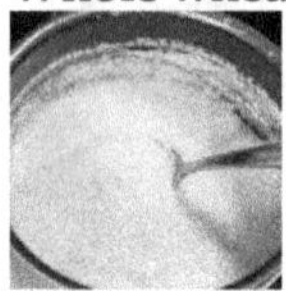

VEGETABLES

Vegetables are vital to the group A diet, providing minerals, enzymes, and anti-oxidants. Eat your vegetables in as natural state as possible. (Raw or steamed) to preserve their full benefits. Most vegetables are available to Group A, but there are a few caveats: peppers aggravate the delicate Group A stomach, as do the molds in fermented olives. Group A is also very sensitive to the lectins in domestic potatoes, sweet potatoes, yarns, and cabbage. Avoid tomatoes, as their lectins have a strongly deleterious effect on the Group A digestive tract.

Some natural Vegetables for group A

Corn   Cucumber

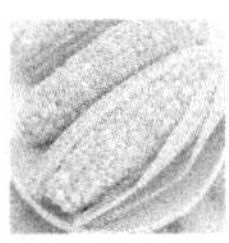 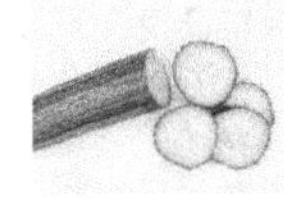

Some beneficial Vegetables for group A

Okra   Lettuce   Onion   Sweet potato

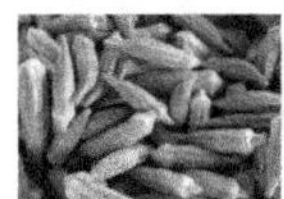 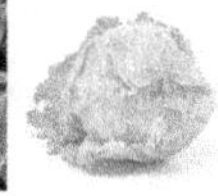 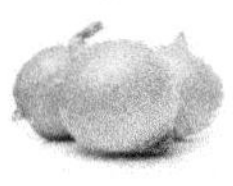 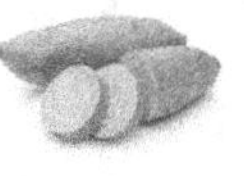

Spinach   Ginger   Pumpkin

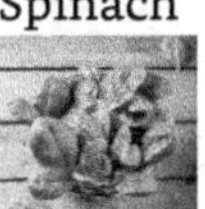 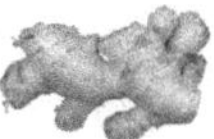 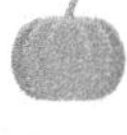

Some detrimental Vegetables for group A

Tomato   Eggplant   Mushroom

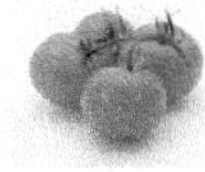 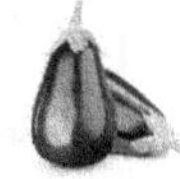 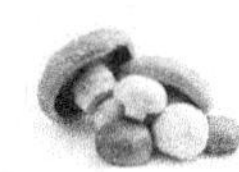

Cabbage   Yam   Chili pepper

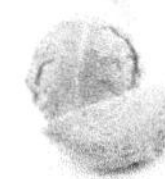 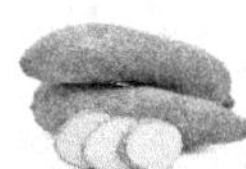 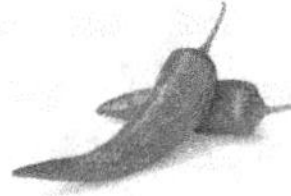

FRUITS

Group A should eat fruits three times a day. Most fruits are allowable, although you should try to emphasize the more alkaline ones, such as berries and plumes, which can help to balance the grains that are acid forming in your muscle tissues. Melons are also alkaline, but their high mod counts make them hard for Group A to digest. Group A doesn't do well on tropical fruits such as mangoes and papaya. Although these fruits contain digestive enzyme that is good for the other blood groups. it doesn't work in group A digestive tract Pineapple on the other hand is an excellent digestive aid for group A. Orange also should be avoided

Oranges are stomach irritant for group A, and they also interfere with the absorption of important mineral.

Some natural fruits for group A

Apple   Melon   Avocado

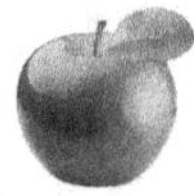 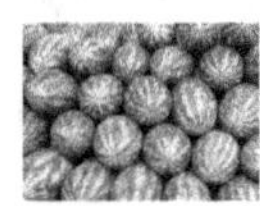 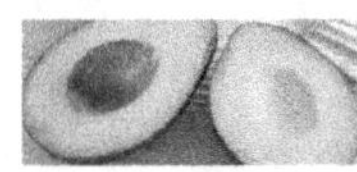

Some beneficial fruits for group A

Pineapple   Lemon   Cherry

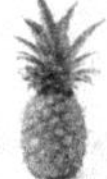 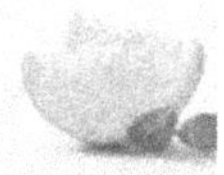 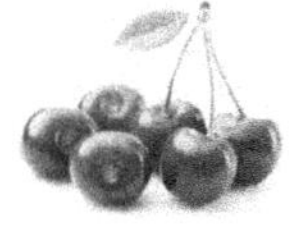

Some detrimental fruits for group A

Pawpaw   Coconut   Banana   Plantain

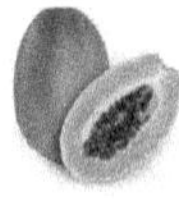 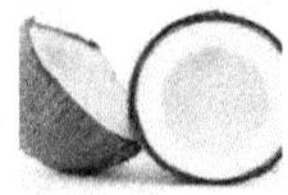 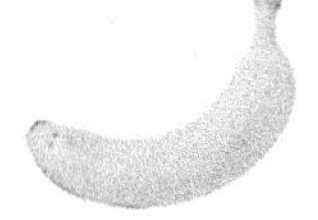 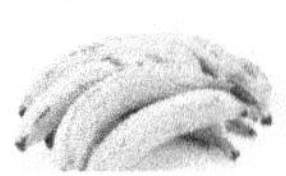

JUICES AND FLUIDS

Group A should start every day with a small glass of warm water into which they have squeezed the juice of one-half lemon. This will help you reduce the mucus that has accumulated overnight in the more sluggish Group A digestive tract and stimulate normal elimination.

Some natural juices and fluids for group A

Apple juice   Cucumber juice

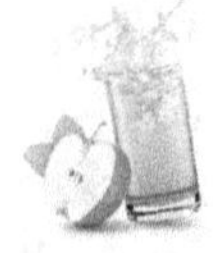 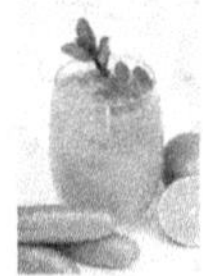

Some beneficial juices and fluids for group A

Aloe juice   Grape juice   Carrot juice

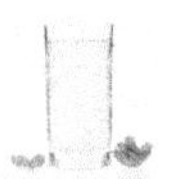

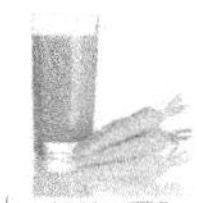

Lemon juice   Pineapple   Black berry

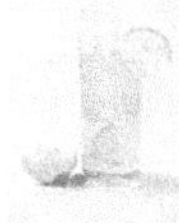

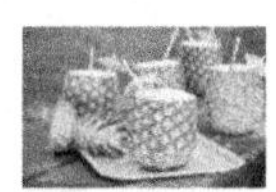

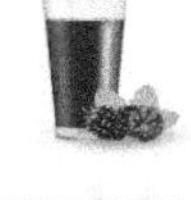

Some detrimental juices and fluids for group A

Coconut milk juice   Cabbage juice   orange juice

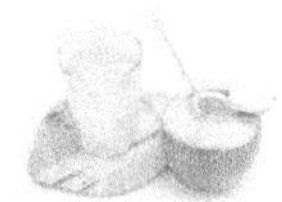

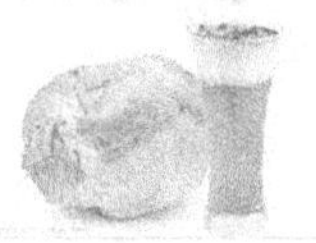

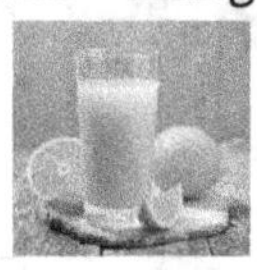

Tangerine juice   Mango juice   Papaya juice

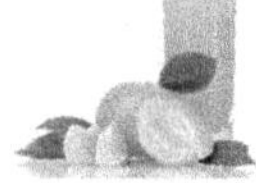

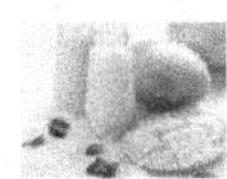

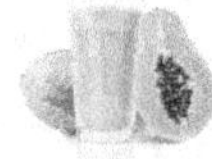

SPICES, SUGARS AND SEASONINGS

Group A should view spices as more than just flavor enchanters. The right combination of spices can be powerful immune-system boosters. For example, soy-based spices such as tamari, miso, and soy sauce are tremendously beneficial for group A. If you are concerned about sodium intake, all of these products are available in low sodium versions. Sugar and chocolate are allowed on the group A diet but only in very small amounts.

Some natural spices, sugars and seasonings for group A

Bay leaf   Honey   Salt

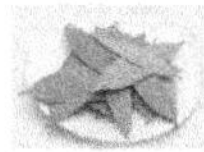

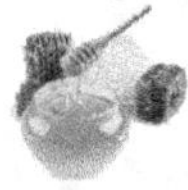

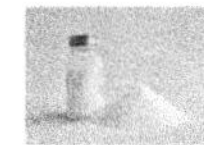

Sugar   Nutmeg

 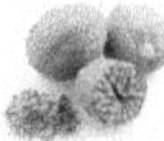

Some beneficial spices, sugars and seasonings for group A

Ginger

Garlic

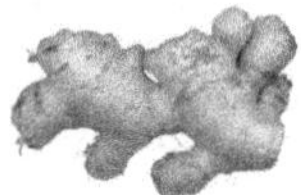 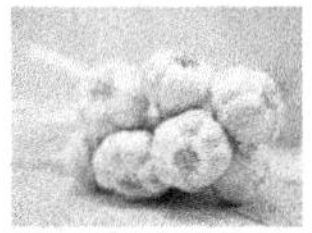

Some detrimental spices, sugars and seasonings for group A

Vinegar

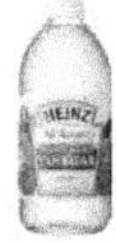

CONDIMENTS

Condiments are not recommended for any blood group. Group A in particular should avoid products with pickles or vinegar because of their low levels of stomach acid.

Some natural Condiments for group A

Apple butter   jam jelly

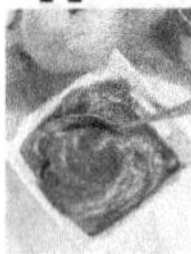 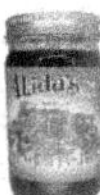

Some beneficial Condiments for group A

Wheat-free soy sauce

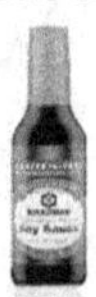

Some detrimental Condiments for group A

Ketchup   mayonnaise

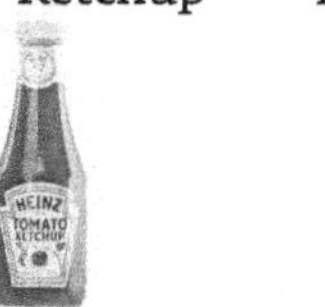
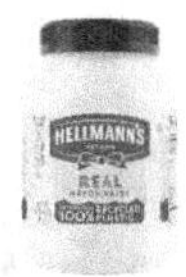

BEVERAGES

Red wine is good for Group A because of its positive cardiovascular effects. A glass of red wine every day is believed to lower the risk of heart disease for both men and women. Coffee may actually be good for group A. All other beverages should be avoided.

Some natural beans for group A

White wine

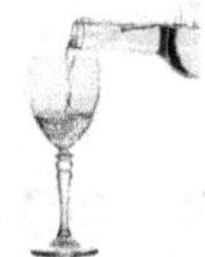

Some beneficial beans for group A

Red wine   green tea   herbal tea   coffee

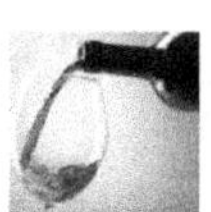
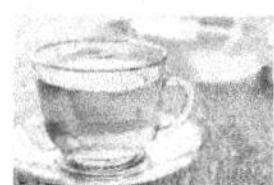
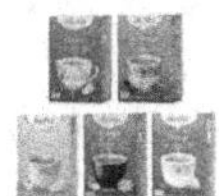
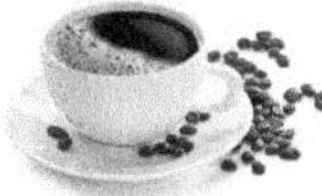

Some detrimental beans for group A

Black tea   beer   soda (club/cola)

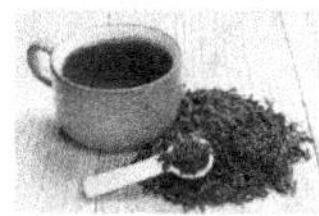
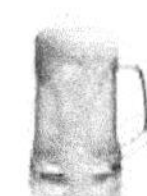
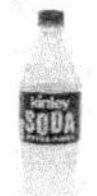

CHAPTER FIVE

BLOOD GROUP B FOOD

The Group B Diet is balanced and wholesome, including a wide variety of foods. The diet should be based on eggs, green leafy vegetables, low-fat dairy and certain meats. This blood group should avoid wheat, corn, lentils, tomatoes and peanuts. Think of B as standing for balance-the balancing forces of A and O. The group also divides foods in three forms, beneficial neutral and detrimental. Beneficial foods act like medicine, neutral foods neither benefit nor harm while detrimental foods act like poison in the body.

FOOD THAT PROMOTES WHEIGT LOSS FOR GROUP B

DAIRY FOODS counters hypoglycemia

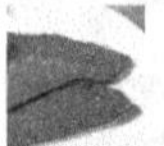

GREEN VEGETABLE aid efficient metabolism

LIVER aid efficient metabolism

MEAT aid efficient metabolism

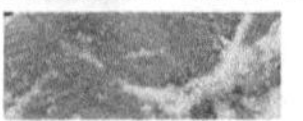

EGGS/LOW FAT aid efficient metabolism

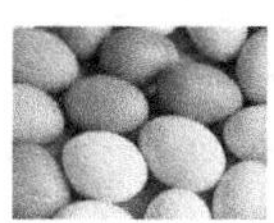

FOOD THAT PROMOTES WHEIGT GAIN FOR GROUP B

PEANUT hampers metabolic efficiency causes hypoglycemia

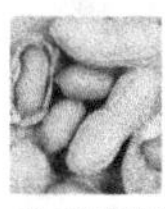

CORN interferes with insulin efficiency, slows metabolic rate

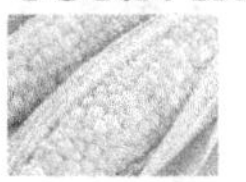

WHEAT cause food to store as fat not burn ads energy

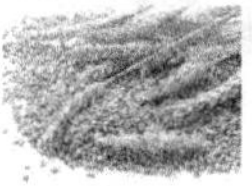

MEAT AND POULTRY

There appears to be a direct connection between stress, and immune disorders, and red meat in the Group B system. That's because your Group B ancestors adapted better to other kinds of meats.

Some natural meat and poultry for group B

Beef   turkey   liver(calf)

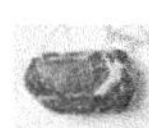 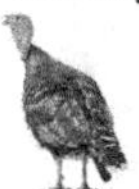 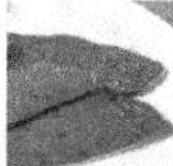

Some beneficial meat and poultry for group B

Lamb   rabbit   goat

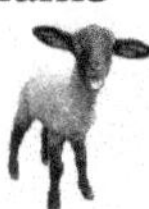 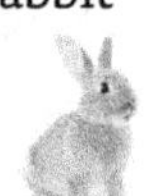 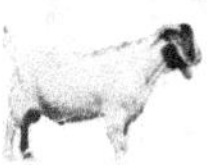

Some detrimental meat and poultry for group B

Pork   duck   turtle quail chicken

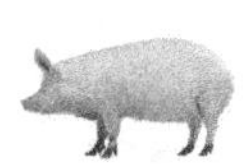 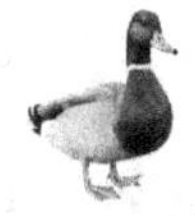 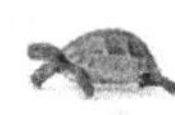

quail   chicken

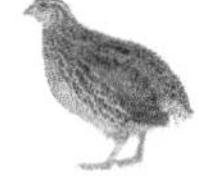 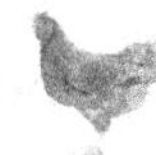

SEA FOODS

Group B thrive on seafood, especially deep-ocean fish such as cod and salmon, which are rich in Nutritious oils. Shell fish such as crab, shrimps, etc. are poorly digested by group B and should be avoided.

Some natural sea foods for group B

Sword fish   cat fish

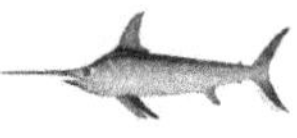 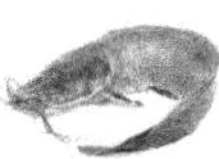

tilapia   red snapper

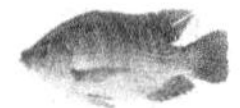 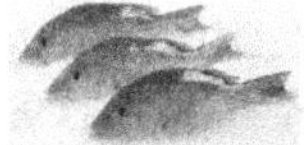

Some beneficial sea foods for group B

Croaker   sardine

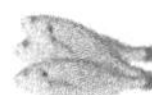 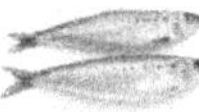

Salmon   white fish

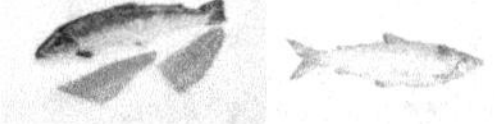

Some detrimental sea foods for group B

Crab   snail   crayfish

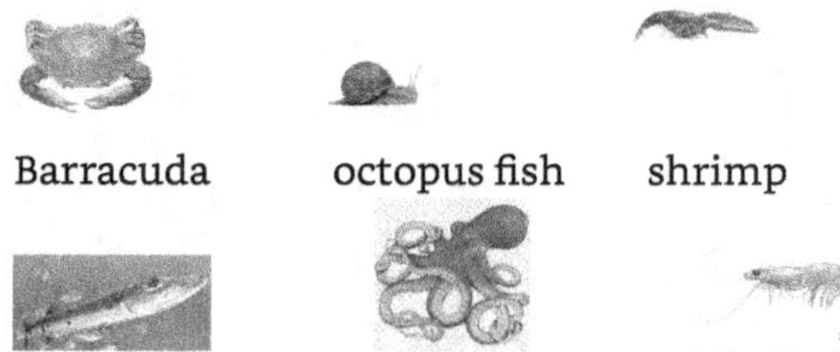

Barracuda   octopus fish   shrimp

DAIRY AND EGGS

Group B is the only blood group that can fully enjoy a variety of dairy foods. That's because the primary sugar in the group B antigen is the very same sugar present in milk. Dairy foods were first introduced to the human diet during the height of group B development by the domestication of animals.

Some natural Dairy and eggs for group B

Butter   egg(chicken)

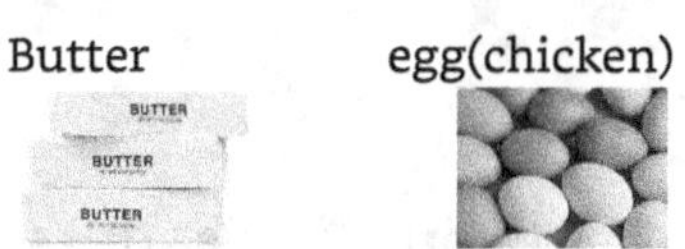

Some beneficial Dairy and eggs for group B

Yogurt   goat milk   cow milk

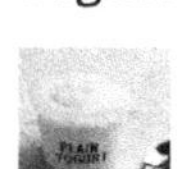 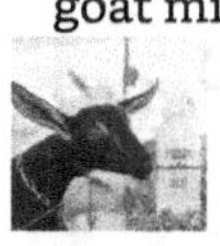 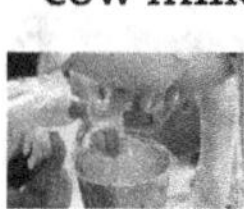

Some detrimental Dairy and eggs for group B

Duck egg   quail egg

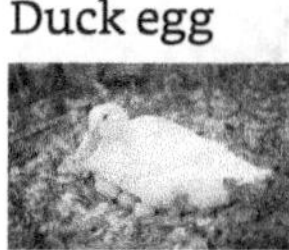 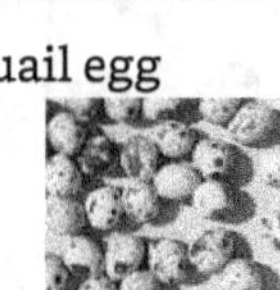

OILS AND FATS

Group B responds well to olive oil. Olive oils encourage proper digestion and healthy elimination. Use at least one table spoon every other day.

Some natural oil and fats for group B

Walnut oil 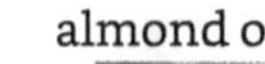 almond oil 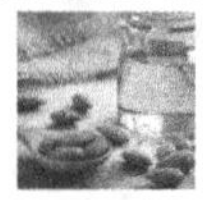 cod liver oil 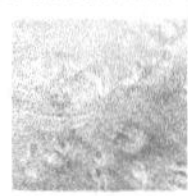

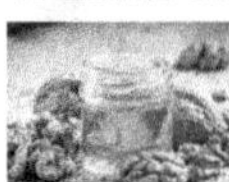

Some beneficial oil and fats for group B

Olive oil

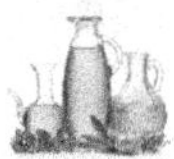

Some detrimental oil and fats for group B

Coconut oil 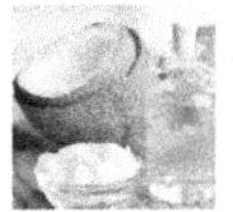 avocado oil 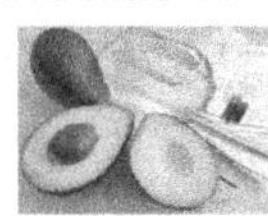

NUTS AND SEEDS

Most nuts and seeds are not advisable for Group B. Peanuts, sesame seeds and sunflower seeds, among others contain lectins that interfere Group B insulin production.

Some natural nuts and seeds for group B

Almond 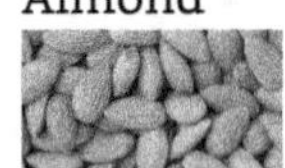 chestnut 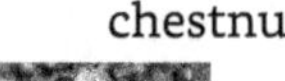 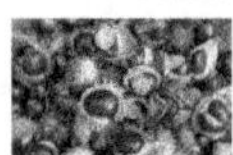

Some beneficial nuts and seeds for group B

Walnut

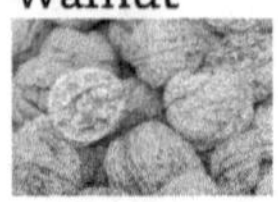

Some detrimental nuts and seeds for group B

Peanut  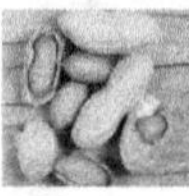 cashew nut 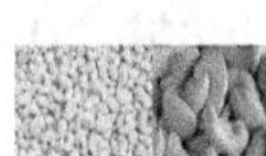

Pumpkin seed   sesame seed

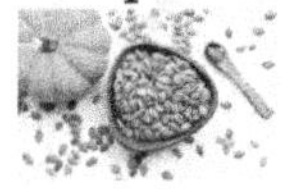
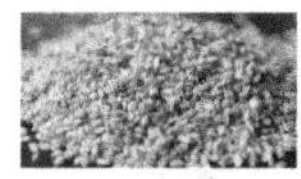

BEANS AND LEGUME

Group B can eat some beans and legumes, but many beans, such as lentils, garbanzos, pintos, and black eye peas, contain lectins that interfere with the production of insulin.

Some natural beans and legume for group B

Fava (broad) beans

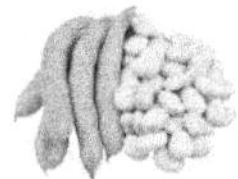

Some beneficial beans and legume for group B

Kidney beans

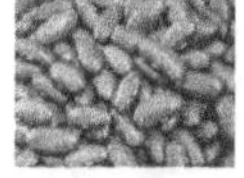

Some detrimental beans and legume for group B

Black eye beans   soy beans

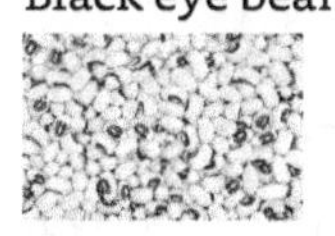
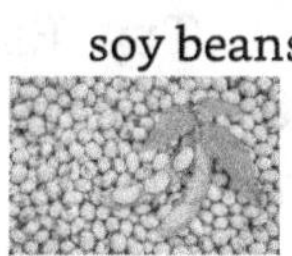

CEREALS

Corn and buckwheat are major factors in Group B weight gain, more than any other food. They contribute to a sluggish metabolism, insulin irregularity, fluid retention, and fatigue. Again, for group B, the key is balance. Eat a variety of grains and cereals. Rice and oats are excellent choices.

Wheat is not tolerated well by most Group B. Wheat contains a lectin that attaches to the insulin receptors in the fat cells, prohibiting insulin from attaching. The result is reduced insulin efficiency and failure to stimulate fat "burning.

Some natural cereals for group B

Cream of rice

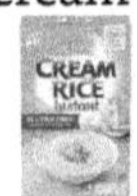

Some beneficial cereals for group B

Millet   oat meal   oat bran

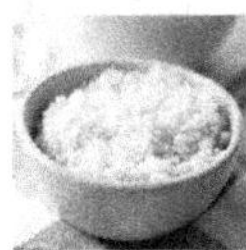 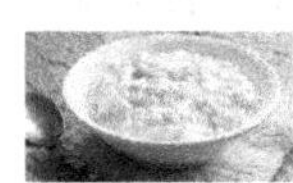 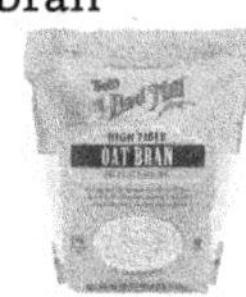

Some detrimental cereals for group B

Corn flakes   tapioca

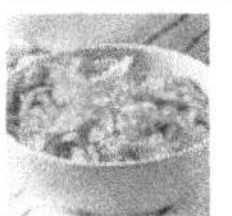 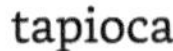 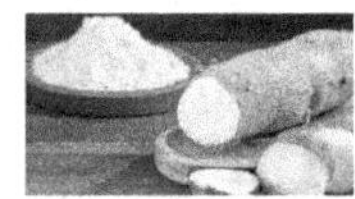

BREAD AND MUFFINS

The recommendations here are similar to those for cereals. Avoid wheat, corn, buckwheat, and rye. That still leaves you a wide variety of breads to choose from. Try Essene or Ezekiel bread, found in health food stores. These live breads are highly nutritious. Although they are sprouted wheat breads, the problem kernel is destroyed. In the sprouting process and they are perfectly helpful.

Some natural bread and muffins for group B

white bread

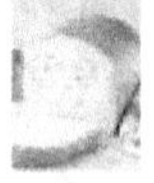

Some beneficial bread and muffins for group B

Brown rice bread   Essen (manna) bread

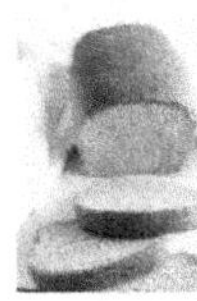 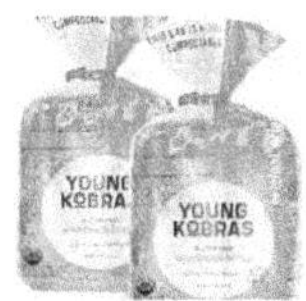

Some detrimental bread and muffins for group B

Wheat bread

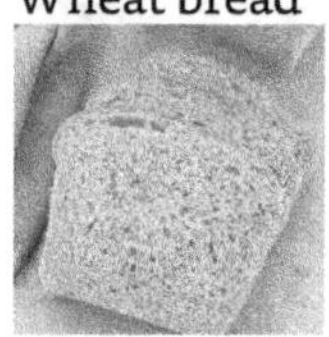

GRAINS AND PASTA

The Group B grain and pasta choices are absolutely consistent with the cereal and bread recommendations. You are however advised that you moderate your intake of pasta and rice.

Some natural grains and pasta for group B

Noodles   rice semolina pasta

Some beneficial grains and pasta for group B

Rice flour oat flour

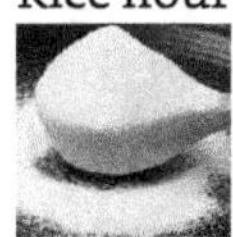 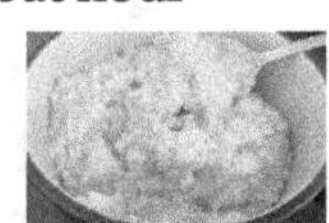

Some detrimental grains and pasta for group B

Durum wheat

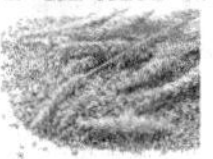

VEGETABLES

There are many high quality, nutritious, group B friendly vegetables, so take full Advantage with three m five servings a day. There are only a handful of vegetables that Group B should avoid, but take these guidelines to heart. Eliminate tomatoes completely from your diet. Tomato is a vegetable called a Solanum Lycopersicon. That means it contains lectins that can agglutinate your blood Group. While the tomato lectin has little effect on group O or group AB. Both group B and group A suffer strong reactions usually in the form of irritation of the stomach lining. Corn is also off your list as it contains those insulin and metabolism-upsetting lectins mentioned before. Since group B tend to be more vulnerable to viruses and auto immune diseases, eat plenty of leafy green vegetables, which contain magnesium, an important antiviral agent.

Some natural vegetables for group B

Garlic   cucumber   spinach   lettuce

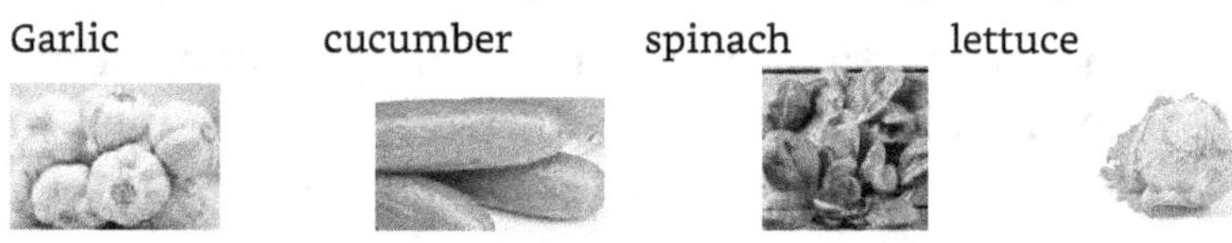

Some beneficial vegetables for group B

Eggplant   cabbage   carrot   ginger

Sweet potato   yam   pepper

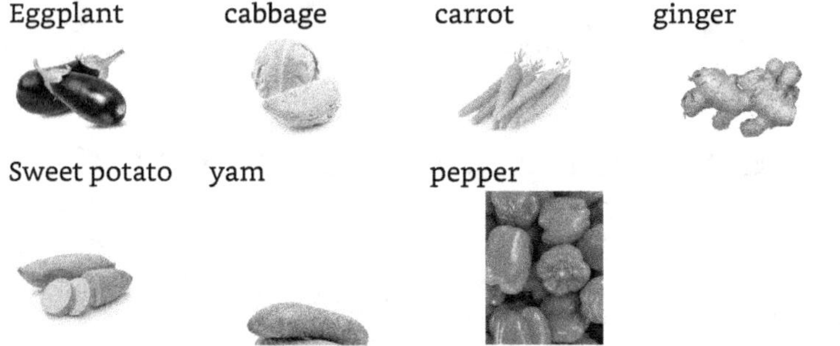

Some detrimental vegetables for group B

Tomato   pumpkin   corn

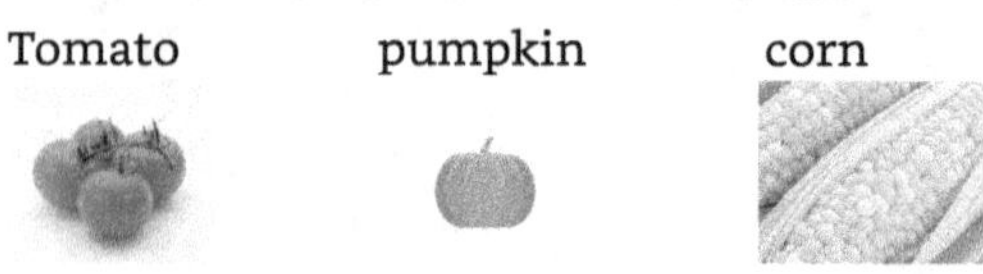

FRUITS

Group B tend to have very balanced digestive systems, with a healthy acid. Alkaline level, so you may have some of the fruits that are too acidic for other blood Groups. Try to incorporate at least one or two fruits from the beneficial list every day to take the advantage of their pro-B medicinal qualities.

Some natural fruits for group B

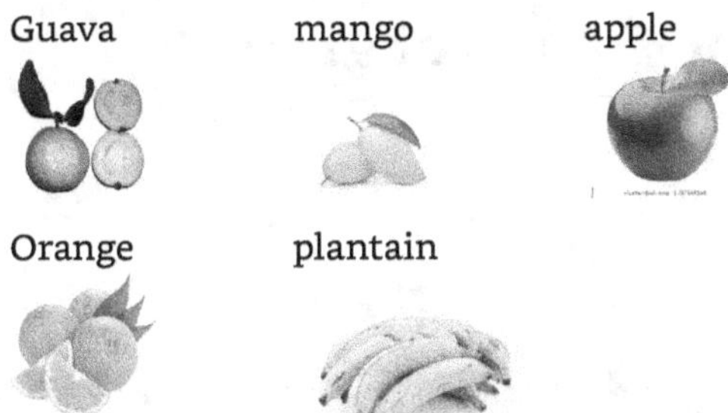

Guava   mango   apple

Orange   plantain

Some beneficial fruits for group B

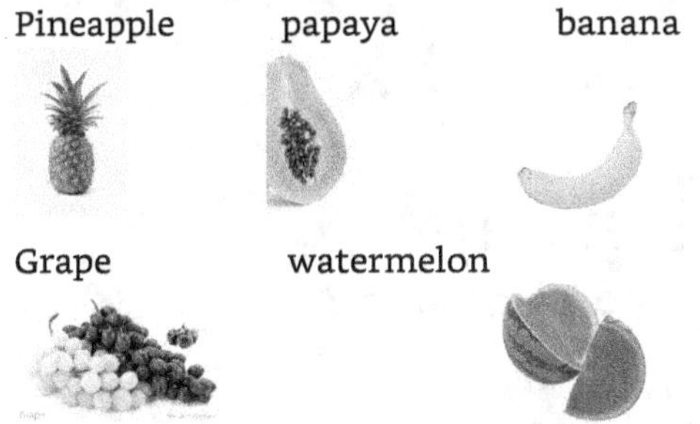

Pineapple   papaya   banana

Grape   watermelon

Some detrimental fruits for group B

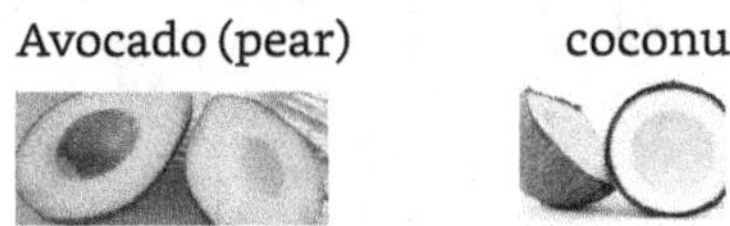

Avocado (pear)   coconut

SPICES, SUGAR AND SEASONINGS

Group B do best with warming herbs, such as ginger, curry, and cayenne pepper. The exceptions are white and black pepper, which contain problem lectins on the reverse side, sweet herbs, tend to be stomach irritants, so avoid barley malt sweeteners, corn syrup, corn starch and cinnamon.

Some natural spices and sugar for group B

Kelp   bay leaf   sugar   salt

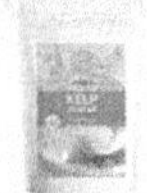 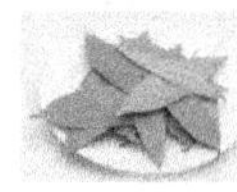 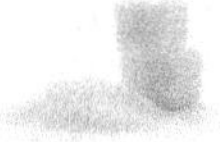 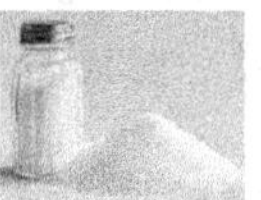

Some beneficial spices and sugar for group B

Curry   ginger

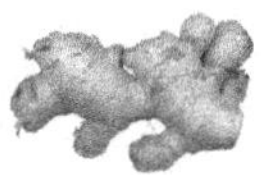

Some detrimental spices and sugar for group B

Corn syrup   aspartame   MSG

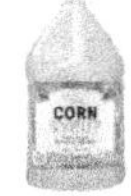 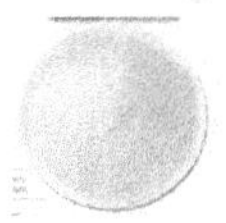 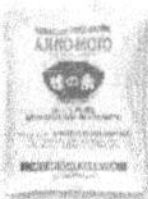

JUICES AND FLUIDS

Most fruit and vegetable juices are good for group B

Some natural juices for group B

Tangerine juice   orange juice   guava juice

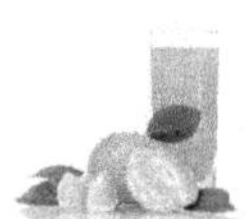 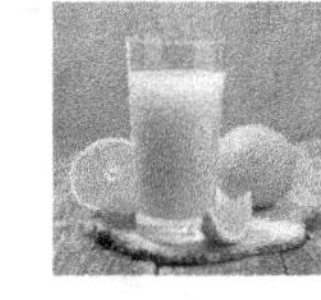 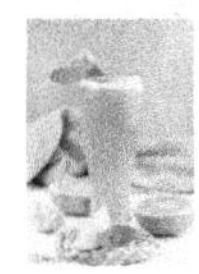

Lemon juice   mango juice   apple juice

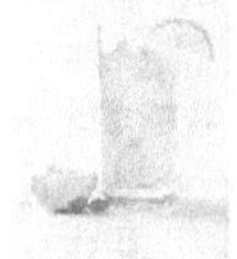 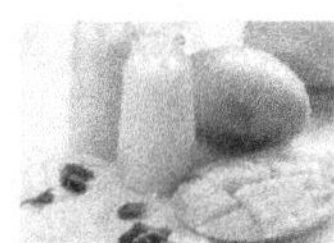

Some beneficial juices for group B

Pineapple juice papaya juice   grape juice

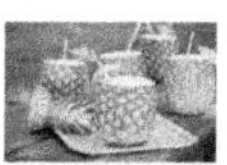 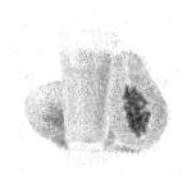 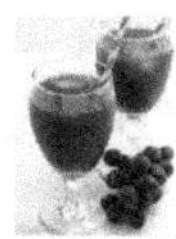

Watermelon juice   banana juice

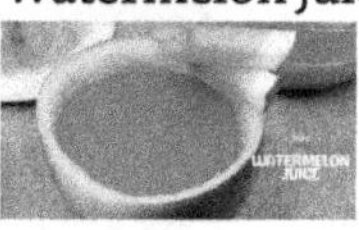 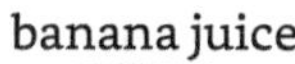 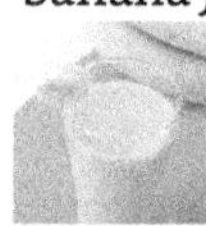

Some detrimental juices for group B

Coconut juice   avocado juice

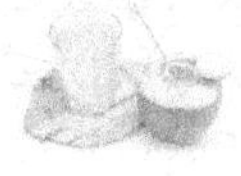 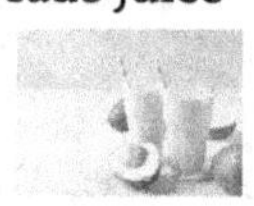

CONDIMENTS

Condiments are basically either neutral or bad for all groups. Group B can handle just about every common condiment except ketchup. (With its dangerous tomato lectins) but common nutritional sense would suggest that you limit your intake of foods that provide no real benefit.

Some natural Condiments for group B

Pickle relish   mayonnaise

 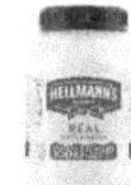

Jam jelly   apple butter

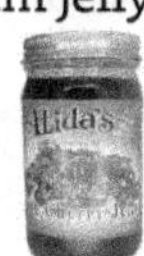 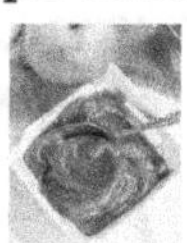

Some beneficial Condiments for group B

Horseradish   cayenne pepper

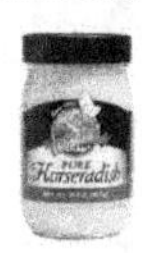 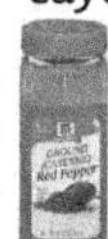

Some detrimental Condiments for group B

Soy sauce   ketchup

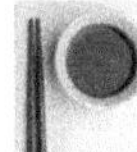
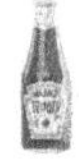

BEVERAGES

Group B do best when they limit their beverages to herbal and green teas, Water, and juice. Although beverages like coffee, regular tea, and wine do no really harm, the goal of the Blood Group Food is to maximize your performance, not to keep it in neutral. If you are a caffeinated coffee or tea drinker, try replacing these beverages with green tea, which has caffeine but also provides some antioxidant benefits.

Some natural beverages for group B

Black tea   coffee (decaf/regular)

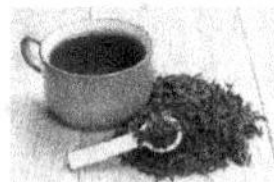
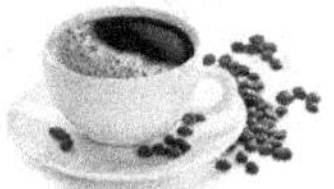

Some beneficial beverages for group B

Green tea   herbal teas

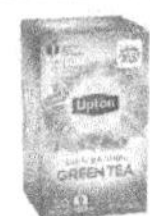
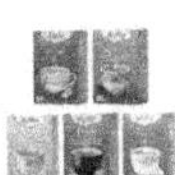

Some detrimental beverages for group B

Seltzer water   liquor   soda (cola/ club)

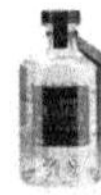
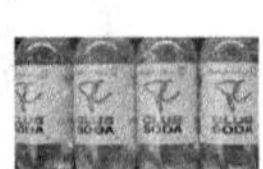

CHAPTER SIX

BLOOD GROUP O FOOD

All groups O thrive on meat and intense physical   activity- the inheritance of their war like hunters' ancestors. This blood group should follow a diet that is high protein, heavy on lean meat, vegetables, fish and poultry. It is okay to skip grains, brans and dairy. Blood group O food like other blood groups food is divided into fifteen groups. Each of these groups divides food into three forms: beneficial. Neutral and detrimental beneficial foods are foods that act like medicine. They help fight diseases; neutral foods are eaten for eating sake, they neither benefit nor harm the body system white detrimental food are foods that act like poison in the body. They are the triggers of diseases.

FOOD THAT PROMOTES WHEIGT LOSS FOR GROUP O

Sea food contain iodine increase thyroid hormone production

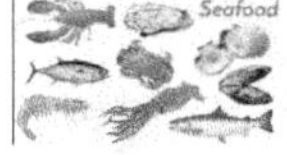

Iodized salt contain iodine, increases thyroid hormone production

Liver B-vitamin source aids efficient metabolism

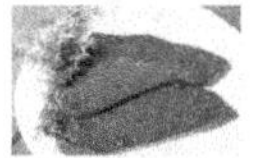

RED MEAT aids efficient metabolism

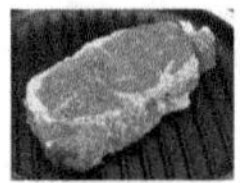

SPINACH aids efficient metabolism

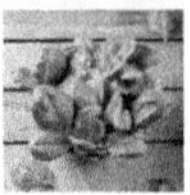

FOOD THAT PROMOTES WHEIGT GAIN FOR GROUP O

WHEAT interfere with insulin efficiency slows metabolic rate

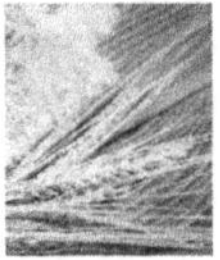

CORN interfere with insulin efficiency slows metabolic rate

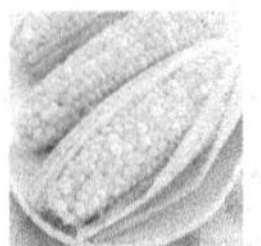

KIDNEY BEAN impairs calorie utilization

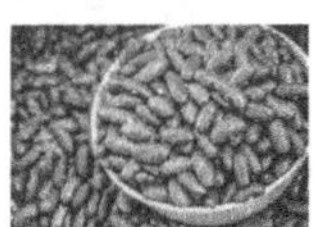

CABBAGE inhibits thyroid hormone

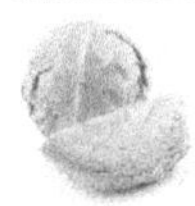

MEAT AND POULTRY

Group O can efficiently digest and metabolize meats because they tend to have high stomach - acid content. This was an essential component in the survival of early Group O

Some natural meat for group o

Turkey   Duck   Chicken

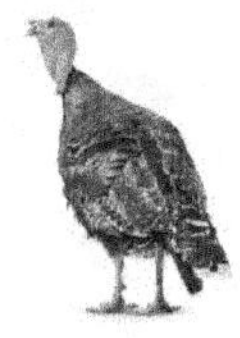 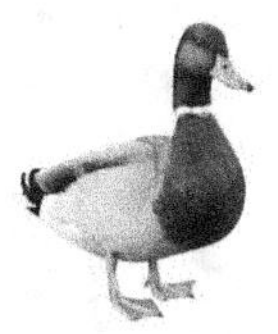 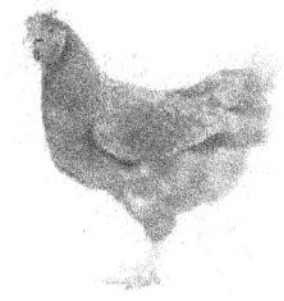

Some beneficial meat for group o

Beef   liver   lamb

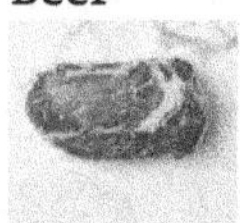 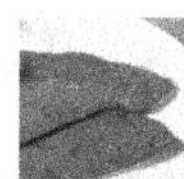 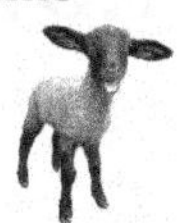

Some detrimental meat for group o

Turtle   Quail   Pork

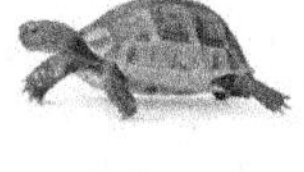 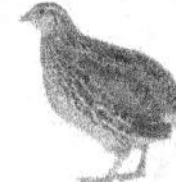 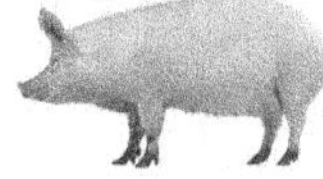

SEA FOODS

Many sea foods are excellent source of iodine, which regulates the thyroid functions. Group O typically have unstable thyroid function which cause metabolic problem and weight gain. Sea food is a major component of the group O diet.

Some neutral sea food for group o

Crab   Shrimp   White fish

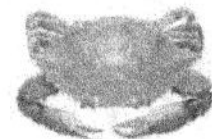 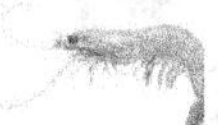 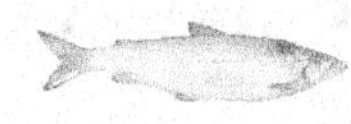

Some beneficial sea food for group o

Tile fish   Sword fish red   snapper fish

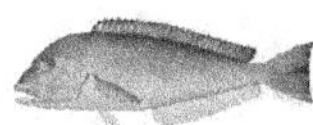 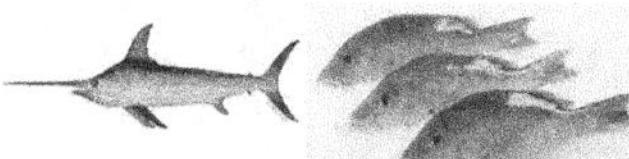

Some detrimental sea food for group o

Octopus fish Cat fish   Barracuda fish

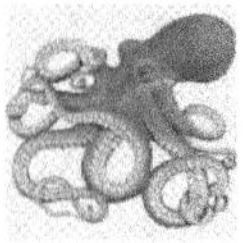 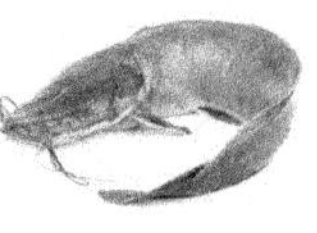 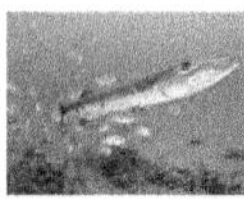

DAIRY AND EGGS

Dairy foods and eggs altogether they tend to be even more difficult for Group O to digest. Soy milk and Soy cheese are excellent high protein alternatives. Ensure to take calcium Supplement. Especially if you are a woman, since dairy foods are the best natural source of absorbable calcium.

Some neutral dairy and egg for group o

Duck egg   Chicken egg

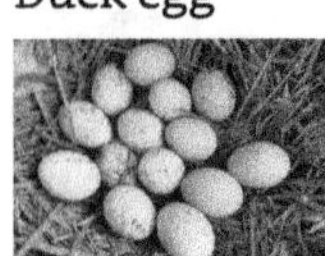 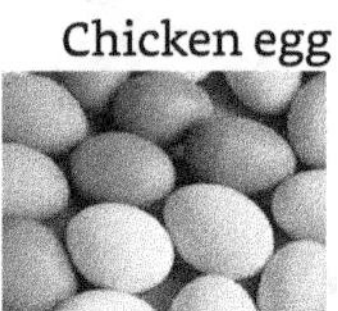

Some beneficial dairy and egg for group o

Soy cheese   Soy milk

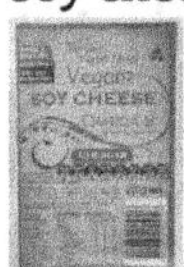 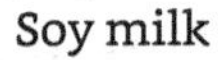 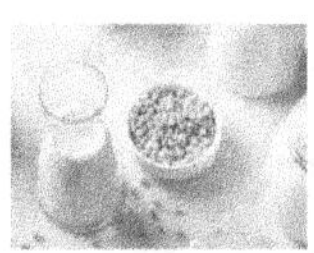

Some detrimental dairy and egg for group o

Cow milk   Goat milk   Quail egg

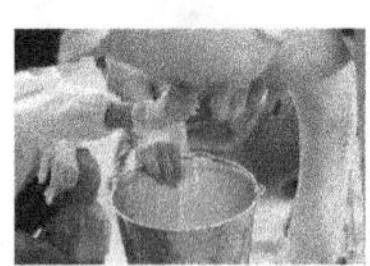 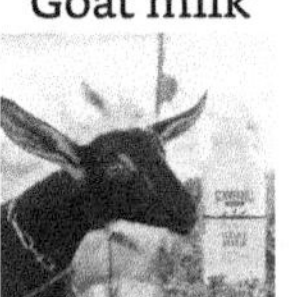 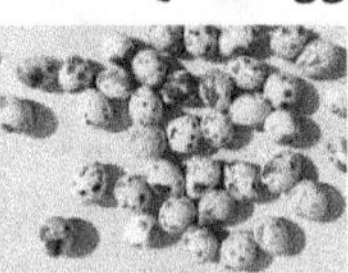

Ice cream

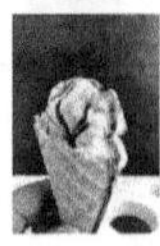

OILS AND FATS

Group O responds well to oils. Oils can be an important source of nutrition and an aid to elimination. Group O should limit their use of oils to the mono-saturated variety, such as olive oil. These oils have Positive effects on the hearts and arteries and may even help reduce blood cholesterol.

Some natural oil for group o

Almond oil

Cod liver oil

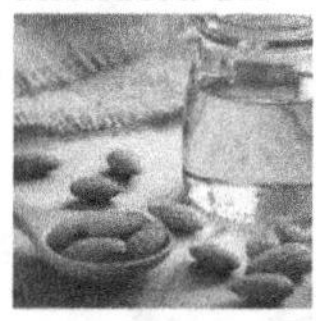

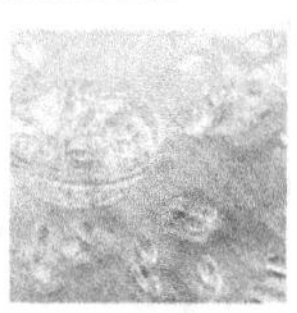

Some beneficial oil for group o

Olive oil

Walnut oil

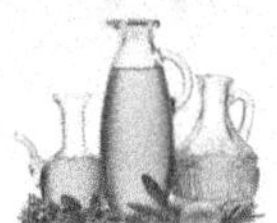

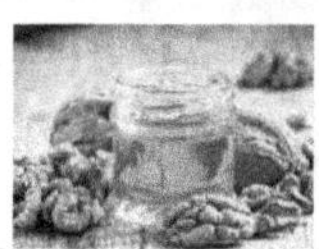

Some detrimental oil for group o

Avocado oil

Coconut oil

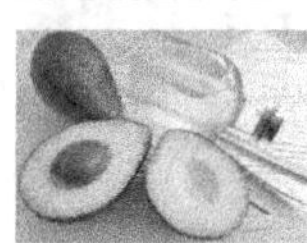

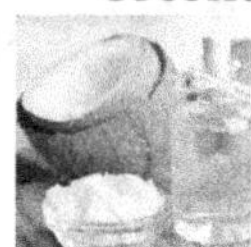

NUTS AND SEEDS

Group O can find a good source of supplemental vegetable protein from some varieties of nuts and seeds. However, these foods should in no way take the place of high-protein meats. Group O certainly doesn't need them in their diet, and should be very selective in their use as they are high in fat. Certainly, one should avoid them if one is trying to lose weight.

Some natural nuts for group o

Almond

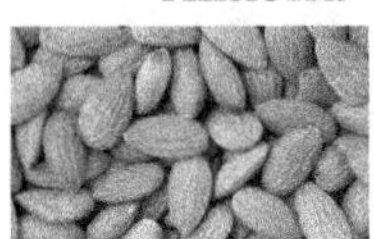

Sesame seed

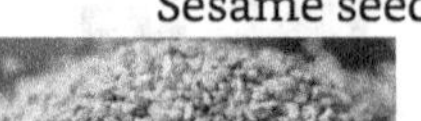

Some beneficial nuts for group o

Pumpkin seed

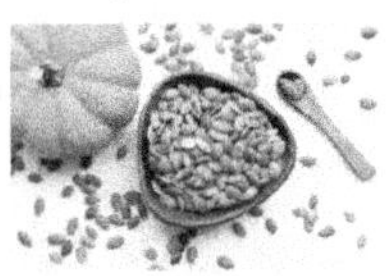

Walnut

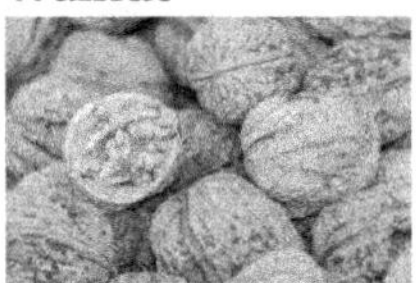

Some detrimental nuts for group o

Chest nut

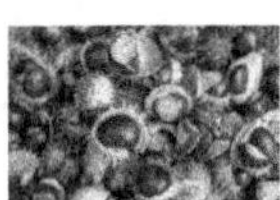

Peanut

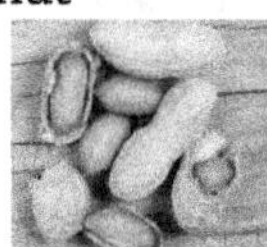

Cashew

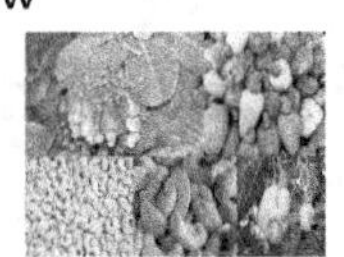

BEANS AND LEGUME

Group O don't utilize beans particularly well; beans inhibit the metabolism of other more important nutrients, such as those found in meat however the few highly beneficial beans are exceptions. They actually promote the strengthening of the digestive tract and prevent ulceration.

Some natural beans for group o

Fava or broad beans

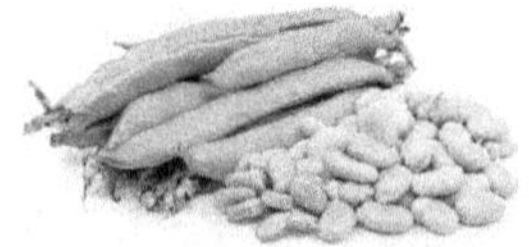

Some beneficial beans for group o

Soy beans   Black-eyed beans

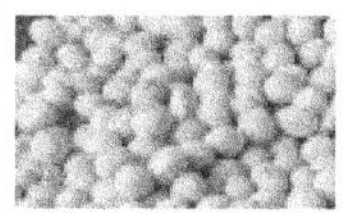 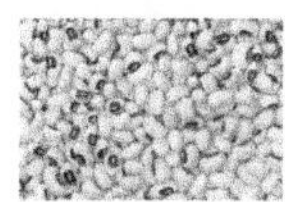

Some detrimental beans for group o

Lentils   Kidney beans

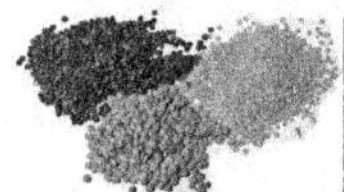 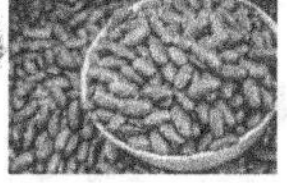

CEREALS

Group O do not tolerate whole wheat products at all and you should eliminate them completely from your diet. They contain lectins that react with both your blood and your digestive tract and interfere with the proper absorption of beneficial foods. Wheat products are a primary culprit in Group 0 weight gain. The gluten in wheat germ interferes with group 0 metabolic processes. Inefficient or sluggish metabolism causes food to convert to energy more slowly and store itself as fat.

Some natural cereals for group o

Oat meal   Millet   Cream of rice

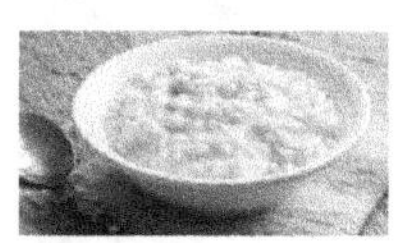 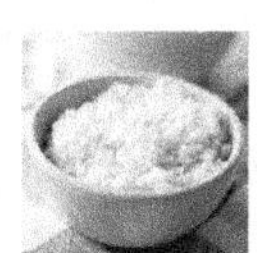 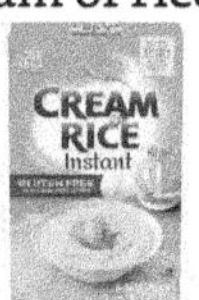

Some beneficial cereals for group o

Buckwheat   rice   kamatz

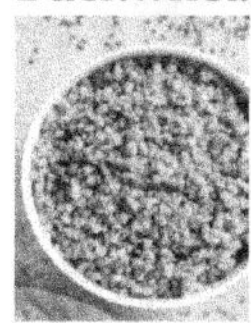 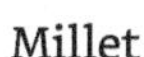 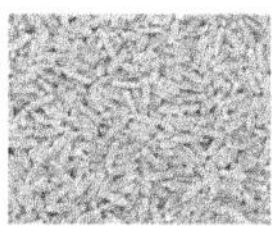

Some detrimental cereals for group o

Cornmeal   Cream of wheat   Cornflakes

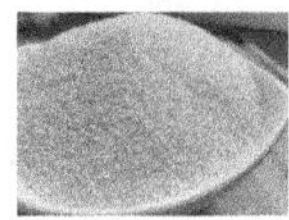 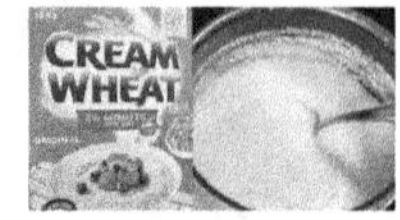 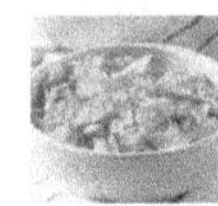

BREAD AND MUFFINS

Obviously, breads and muffins can be a source of trouble for Group O, since most of them contain some wheat. Even. Wheat-free breads can be troublesome for Group O if they eat them often enough their genetic makeup is not assimilated to the consumption of grains. Two exceptions are Essene and Ezekiel bread, which are usually found in the freezer section of your local health food store. These sprouted seed breads are assailable to group O because the gluten lectins (principally found in the seed coats) are destroyed by the sprouting process, unlike commercially produced bread.

Some natural bread for group o

Brown rice bread

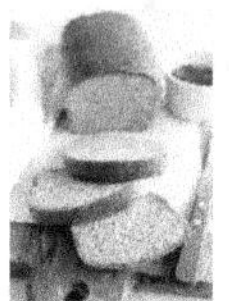

Some beneficial bread for group o

Essene mana bread

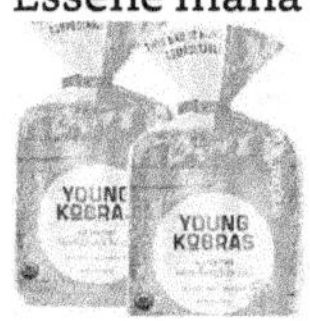

Some detrimental bread for group o

Wheat bread

White bread

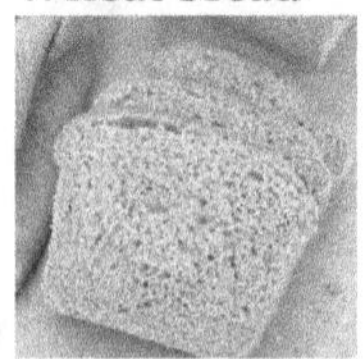 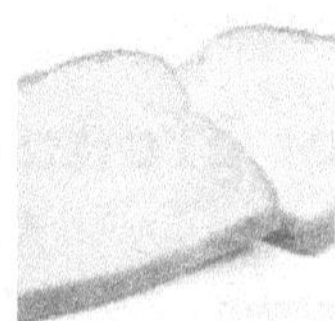

GRAINS AND PASTA

Most pasta is made with semolina wheat, so you'll need to be very careful if you want an occasional pasta dish made from buckwheat. Rice flour is better tolerated by group O.

Some natural grains and pasta for group o

Rice flour 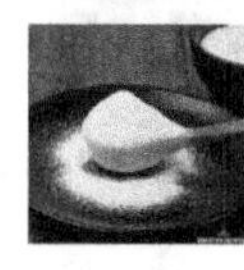   Noddle's 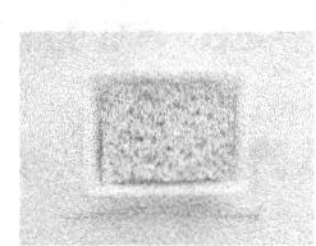   Rice 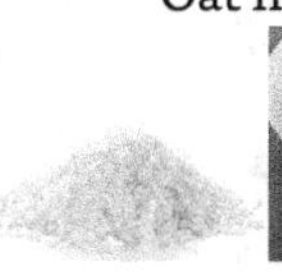   Oat flour 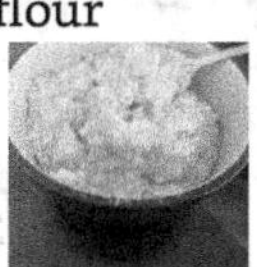

Some beneficial grains and pasta for group o

Buckwheat 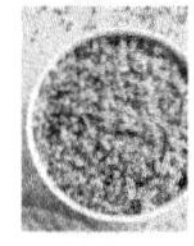   Millet 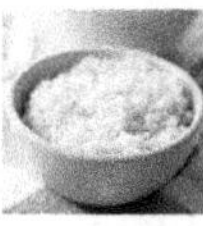

Some detrimental grains and pasta for group o

Semolina pasta 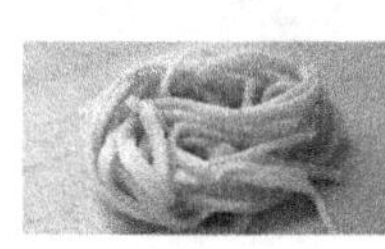   Durum wheat 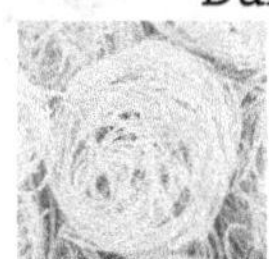

VEGETABLES

There are a tremendous number of vegetables available to Group O, and they form a critical component of your diet, you cannot, however, simply eat all vegetables indiscriminately. Several classes of vegetables cause big problems for Group O.

The molds in domestic mushrooms, as well as fermented olives, tend to trigger allergic reactions in group O. All of these foods are foreign to the group O system which has not designed to handle them. The nightshade vegetables, such as eggplant and potatoes cause arthritic conditions in group O because their lectins deposit in the tissue surrounding the joints.

Corn lectins affect the production of insulin, often leading to diabetes and obesity. All Group O should avoid corn-especially if you have a weight problem or a family history of diabetes. Tomatoes are a special case. Heavily laced with powerful lectins, tomatoes are troubles for group A and B digestive tracts. However, Group Os can eat tomatoes. They become neutral in your system.

Some natural vegetable for group o

Carrot   Yam   Cabbage

Gallic   Tomato

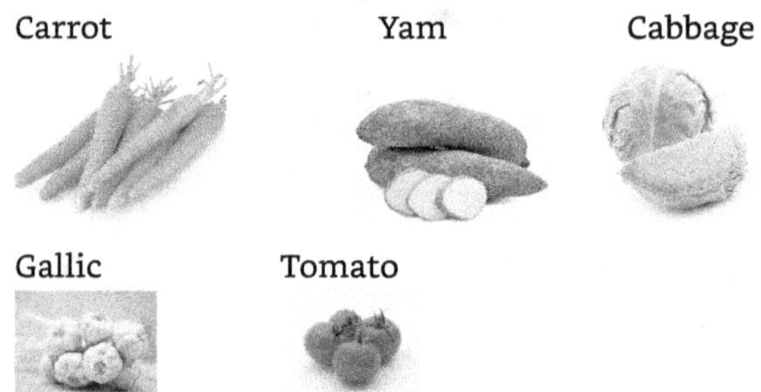

Some beneficial vegetable for group o

Okra   Lettuce   Onion   Sweet potato

Spinach   Ginger   Pumpkin

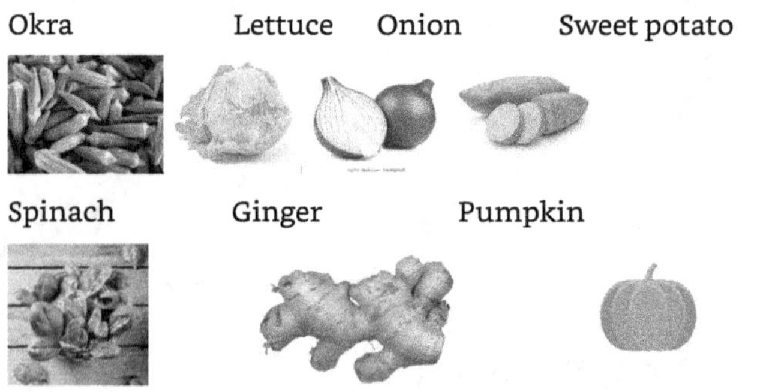

Some detrimental vegetable for group o

Cucumber   Eggplant   Mushroom   corn

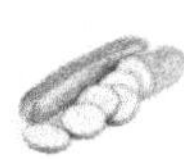 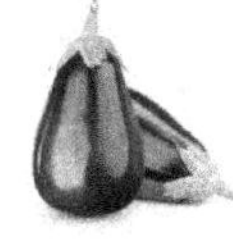 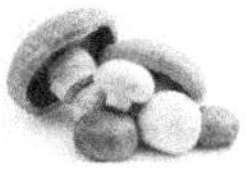 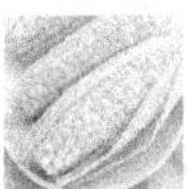

FRUITS

Many wonderful fruits are available on the Group O Diet, Fruits are not only an important source of fiber, vitamins and minerals, but they can be an excellent alternative to bread and pastas for group O if you eat a piece of fruit rather than a slice of bread, your system will be better served at the same time you will be supporting your weight-loss goals. It may surprise you to find same of your favorite fruits on the dangerous list and some add choices on the beneficial lists.

The reason that plums, prunes and figs are so beneficial to your blood group is that most dark red, blue, and purple fruits tend to cause an alkaline rather than an acidic reaction in your digestive tract. The group O digestive tract has high acidity and needs the balance of alkaline to reduce ulcers and irritation of stomach lining. However, just because a fruit is alkaline doesn't mean it is good for you. Melons are also alkaline but they contain high molds counts, to which group O has a proven sensitivity.

Oranges, tangerines, and strawberries should be avoided because of their high acid content. Grapefruit also has a high acid content, but you may eat it in moderation because it exhibits alkaline properties after digestion. Most other berries are okay, but stay away from blackberries which contain a leap that aggravates group O digestion.

Some natural fruits for group o

Grapes   Watermelon   Apple   Pawpaw

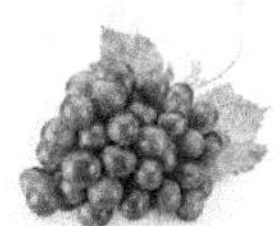 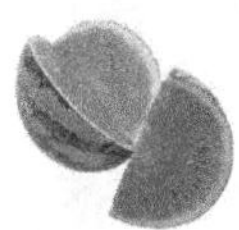 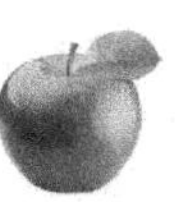 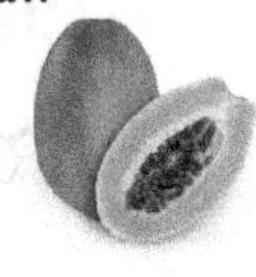

Some beneficial fruits for group o

Mango   Cherry   Banana

Guava   Pineapple

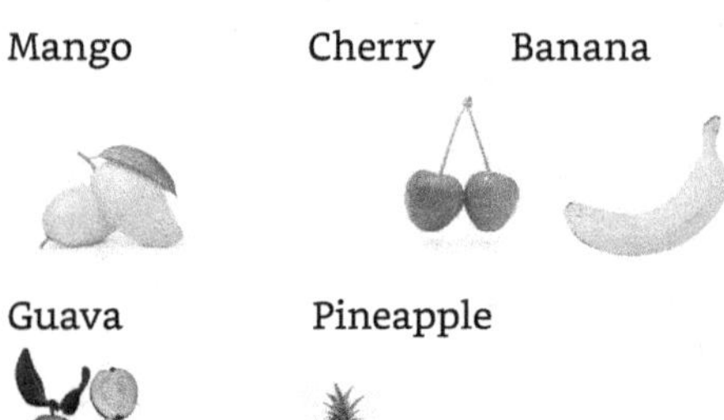

Some detrimental fruits for group o

Coconut   Orange   Plantain

Melon   Tangerine

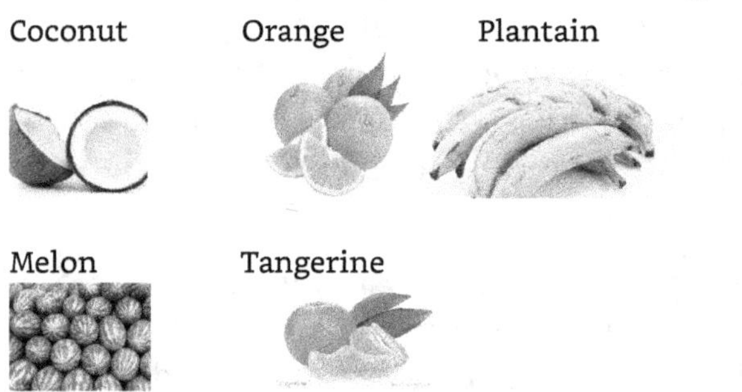

JUICES AND FLUIDS

Vegetable juices are preferable to fruit juices for Group O because of their alkalinity. If you drink fruit juice, choose a low sucrose variety. Avoid high sugar juices such as apple juice. Pineapple juice can be particularly helpful in avoiding water retention and bloating, both factors which contribute to weight gain. Black cherry is also a beneficial alkaline juice.

Some natural juices and fluids for group o

Lemon juice   Grape juice Carrot juice Pawpaw juice

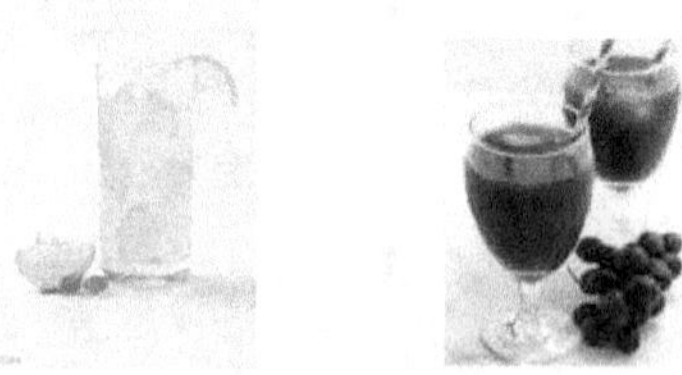

Some beneficial juices and fluids for group o

Black cherry juice   Mango juice   Prune juice

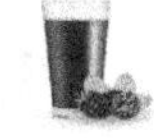
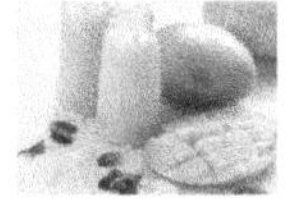
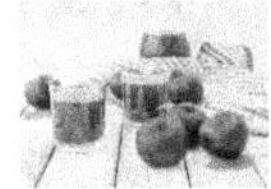

Guava juice   Spinach juice

Some detrimental juices and fluids for group o

Coconut milk   orange juice   Aloe juice

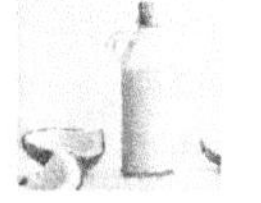
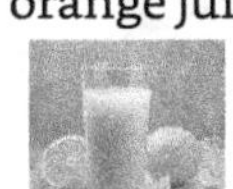
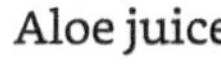

Blackberry juice   Cucumber juice   Tangerine juice

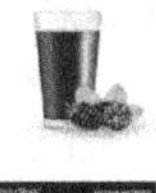
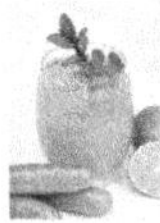
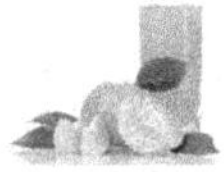

SPICES, SUGAR AND SEASONINGS

Your choice of spices can actually improve your digestive and immune systems. For example, kelp-based seasonings are very good for Group O because they are rich sources of iodine. Iodized salt is another good source of iodine, but use it sparingly. The kelp bladder wrack tends to counter the hyper acidity of the Group O digestive tract, reducing the potential for ulcers. The abundant fructose in the kelp protects the intestinal lining of the group O stomach, preventing ulcer-causing bacteria. Keep in mind also that kelp is highly effective as a metabolic regular for group O, and is an important aid to weight loss.

Parsley is soothing to your digestive tract, as are certain warming spices, like curry and cayenne pepper Note; however, that black and white pepper and vinegar are irritants to the group O stomach. Sugar products such as honey and sugar will not harm you nor will chocolate. But these should all be strictly limited to occasional use as condiments. Avoid corn syrup as a sweetener.

Some natural spices, Sugar and seasonings for group o

Chocolate Sugar Bay leaf Honey

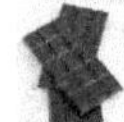  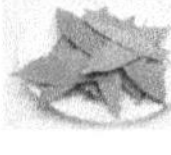 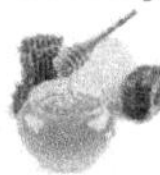

Some beneficial spices, Sugar and seasonings for group o

Kelp Iodized salt Curry

 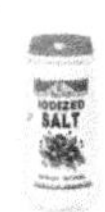

Some detrimental spices, Sugar and seasonings for group o

Aspartame MSG Nutmeg

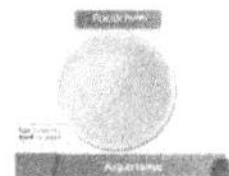  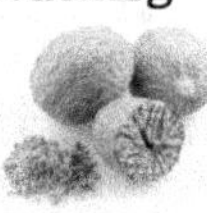

CONDIMENTS

There are no highly beneficial condiments for Group O. If you must have mustard or salad dressing on your foods, use them in moderation, and stick to the low-fat, low-sugar varieties. Although group O can have tomatoes occasionally, avoid ketchup that also contains ingredients like vinegar. All pickled foods are indigestible for group O. They severely irritate the group O stomach lining.

Some natural condiments for group o

Apple butter Soy sauce Jam jelly

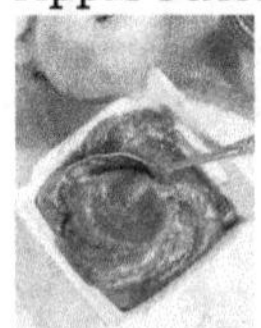 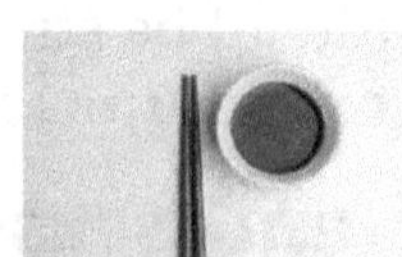 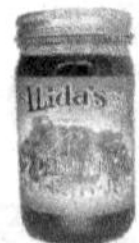

Some beneficial condiments for group o

Carob   curry powder   parsley

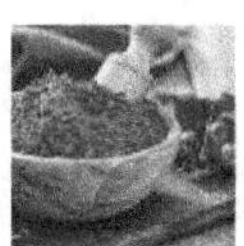
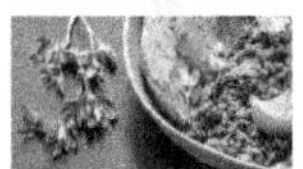

Some detrimental condiments for group o

Pickles relish   Ketchup   Mayonnaise

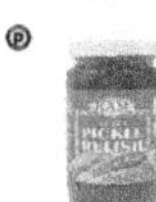
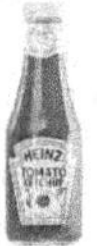
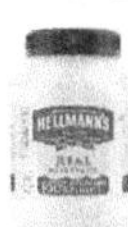

BEVERAGES

There are very few acceptable beverages for group O. You are pretty much limited to the innocuous effect of seltzer, club soda and tea. Wine and beer do not benefit you and could be detrimental to you if not taken in modest quantity and not limited to occasions. Green tea is okay, it is allowed as acceptable substitute for other caffeinated products, but it contains no special curative properties for group O. The problem that coffee poses for group O is in the increased levels of stomach acid it produces. Group O have plenty of stomach acid on their own they really don't need help. IF you a coffee drinker, perhaps you can begin to gradually cut down on the amount you consume each day. Your ultimate goal is to eliminate drinking coffee altogether. The common withdrawal symptoms, such as headache, Fatigue, and irritability, won't occur if you wean yourself gradually.

Some natural beverages for group o

Red wine (moderate)   Beer (moderate)

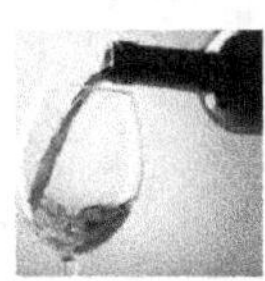
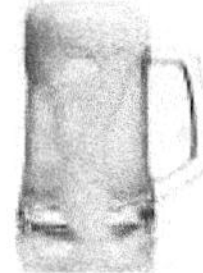

Some beneficial beverages for group o

Seltzer water   Club soda

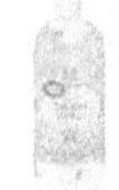

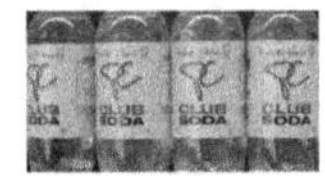

Herbal teas   green teas

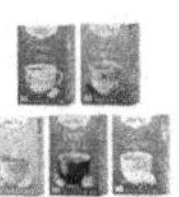

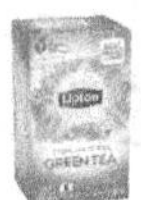

Some detrimental beverages for group o

Block tea   Liquor   Cola

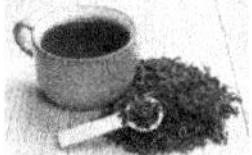

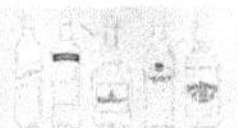

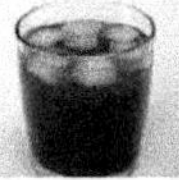

Coffee   Wine (excess)   Beer (excess)

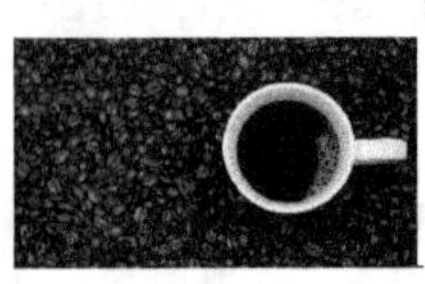

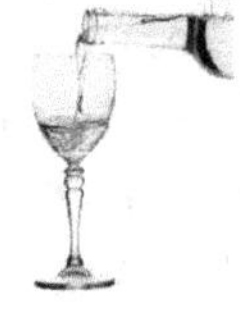

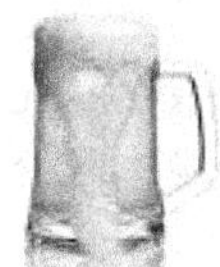

CHAPTER SEVEN

BLOOD GROUP AB FOOD

This group should focus mostly on tofu, seafood, green and leafy vegetables and should avoid caffeine intake, alcohol, smoking cigarettes and cured meats.   The fifteen food groups of AB blood group also divide foods in three forms beneficial, neutral and detrimental. The beneficial foods act like medicine, neutral does neither benefit nor harm, while detrimental foods trigger diseases.

FOOD THAT PROMOTES WHEIGT LOSS FOR GROUP AB

SEA FOODS promotes metabolic efficiency

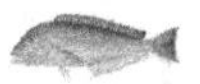

VEGETABLE improves metabolic efficiency

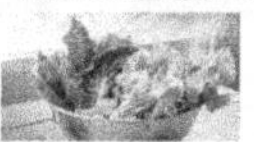

TOFU promotes metabolic efficiency

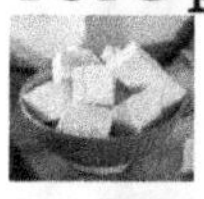

DAIRY FOODS improves insulin production

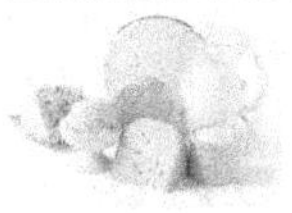

FOOD THAT PROMOTES WHEIGT GAIN FOR GROUP AB

MEAT poorly digests

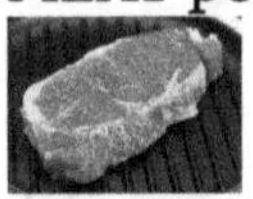

KIDNEY BEANS inactive digestive enzymes, slow metabolic rate

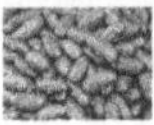

CORN inhabit insulin efficiency

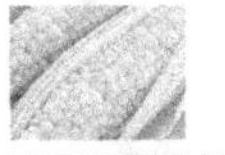

WHEAT IN OVER ABUNDANCE impair calorie utilization

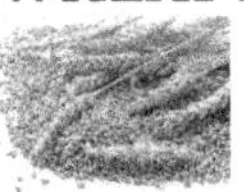

MEATS AND POULTRY

When it comes to eating meat and poultry, group AB borrow characteristics from bath group A and B. Like group A you do not produce enough stomach acid to effectively digest too much animal protein. Yet the key for you is portion size and frequency. Group AB need some meat protein, especially the kinds of meat that represent Your B like heritage lamb, Mutton, rabbit and turkey, instead of beef.

Some natural meat and poultry for group AB

Goat

rabbit

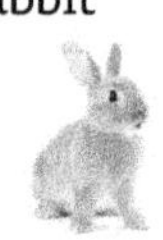

Liver

lamb

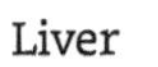

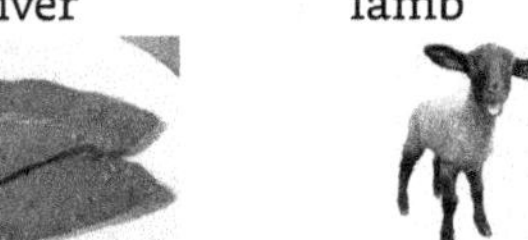

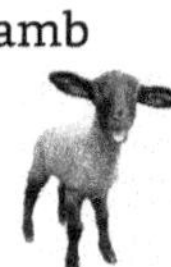

Some beneficial meat and poultry for group AB

Turkey

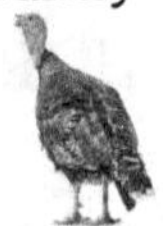

Some detrimental meat and poultry for group AB

Chicken

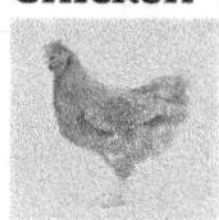

beef

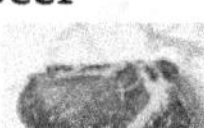

Turtle

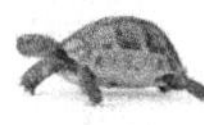

pork

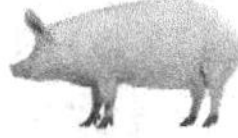

DAIRY AND EGGS

For dairy foods, group AB can put on the "B" hat. You benefit from dairy foods, especially cultured and soured products yogurt, kefir, and non-fat sour cream which are more easily digested. The primary factor you have to watch out for is excessive mucus production. Like group A, you already produce a lot of mucus, and you don't need more. Eggs are a very good source of protein for group AB.

Some natural dairy and eggs for group AB

Cow milk

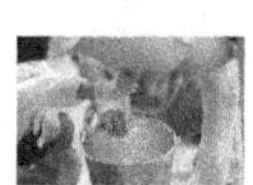

quail egg

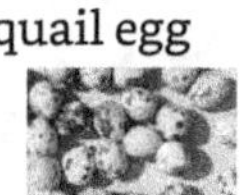

chicken eggs

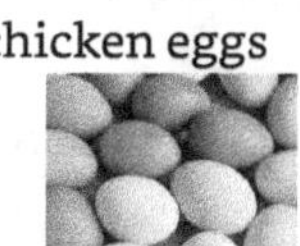

Some beneficial dairy and eggs for group AB

Yogurt

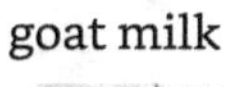

goat milk

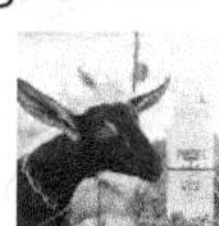

Some detrimental dairy and eggs for group AB

Ice cream

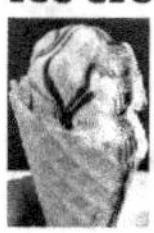

cow milk (whole)

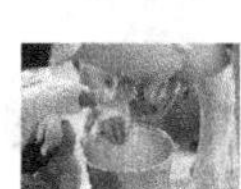

duck egg

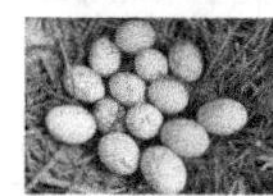

NUTS AND SEEDS

Nuts and seeds present a mixed picture for group AB. Eat them in small amounts and with caution. Although they can be a good supplementary protein source, all seeds contain the insulin inhibiting lectins that make them a problem for Bs. On the other hand, you share the group A preference for peanuts, which are powerful immune boosters.

Some natural Nuts and seeds for group AB

Almond

cashew

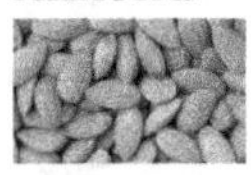
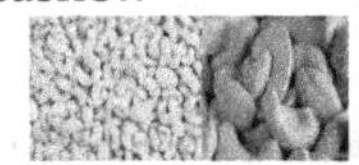

Some beneficial Nuts and seeds for group AB

Peanut

walnut

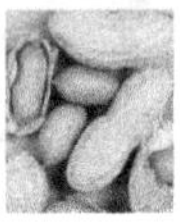
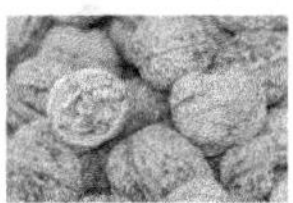

Some detrimental Nuts and seeds for group AB

Sesame seeds

pumpkin seeds

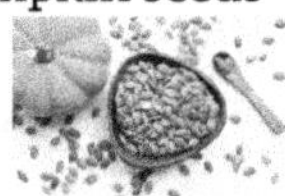

BEANS AND LEGUMES

Beans and legumes are another mixed bag for group AB. For example, lentils beans are an important cancer-fighting food for group AB, although they are not advised for group B, in particular, lentils are known to contain cancer fighting antioxidants. On the other hand, kidney and lima beans, which slow insulin production in Group A, have the same effect in group AB.

Some natural Beans and legumes for group AB

Northern bean

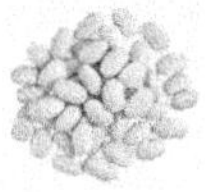

Some beneficial Beans and legumes for group AB

Soy beans   lentils

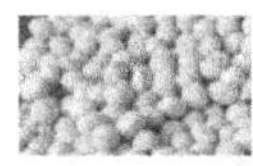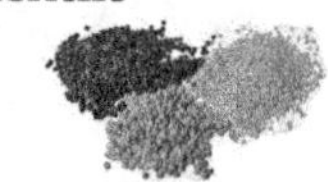

Some detrimental Beans and legumes for group AB

Kidney bean   black eye bean fava (broad) beans

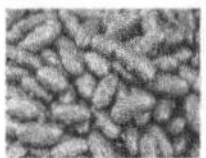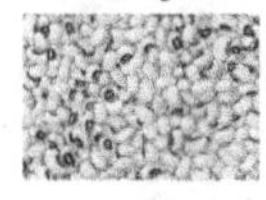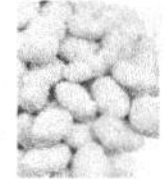

CEREALS

Generally, you do well on grains, even wheat, but need to limit your wheat consumption because the inner kernel for group AB is highly acid forming for group AB. Limit, your intake of wheat germ and bran to once a week. Oatmeal, soy flakes, millet, ground rice and soy granules are good Group AB, but you must avoid buckwheat and com.

Some natural cereals for group AB

Cream of rice

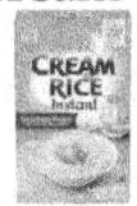

Some beneficial cereals for group AB

Oat meal   millet

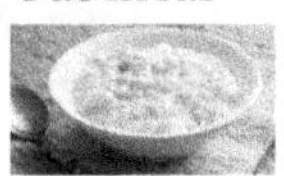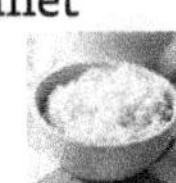

Some detrimental cereals for group AB

Corn meal

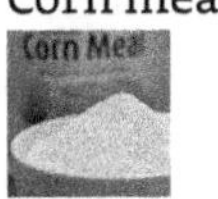

tapioca

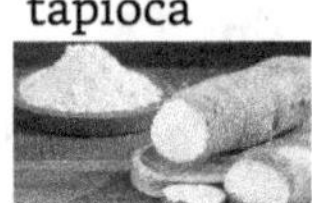

Buck wheat

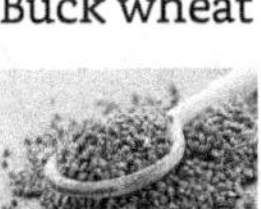

corn flakes

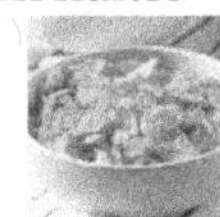

BREADS AND MUFFINS

The Group AB guidelines for breads and muffins are similar to those of cereals and grains. They are generally favorable foods. But if you produce excessive mucus or are overweight, these conditions make whole wheat inadvisable. Soy and rice flour are good substitutes for you.

Some natural bread for group AB

Wheat bread

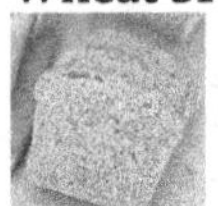

Some beneficial bread for group AB

Brown rice bread

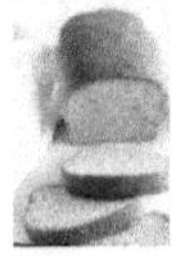

Some detrimental bread for group AB

Corn muffin

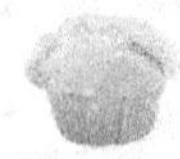

GRAINS AND PASTA

Group AB' benefits from a diet rich in rice rather than pasta, you may have semolina or spinach pasta once or twice a week. Again, avoid com and buckwheat in favor of oats. Limit your intake of bran and wheat germ to once in a week.

Some natural grains and pasta for group AB

Wheat flour 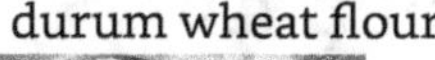 durum wheat flour   semolina pasta

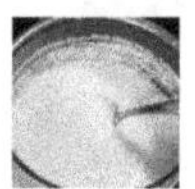 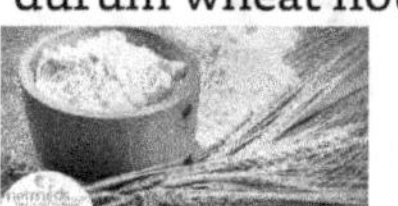 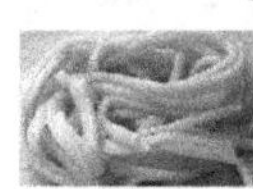

Some beneficial grains and pasta for group AB

Rice   oat flour 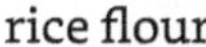 rice flour

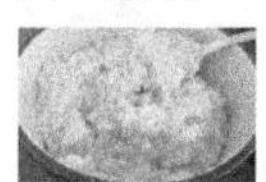 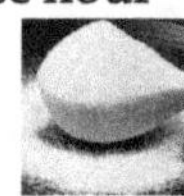

Some detrimental grains and pasta for group AB

Saba noodles   buck wheat flour

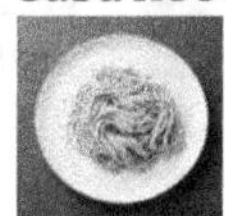 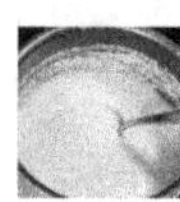

SEA FOODS

Blood type AB does very well with seafood as a matter of fact; there are many different seafood items that are greatly beneficial to their health and wellbeing acting similar to that of medicine. These include cod, grouper, hake, mackerel, mahi-mahi, monkfish, ocean perch, pickerel, pike, porgy, rainbow trout, red snapper, sailfish, salmon, sardines, sea trout, shad, snail, sturgeon, albacore tuna, and yellowtail. On the other hand, there are quite a few seafood items that should be avoided by blood type AB as they poison the body. These include anchovy, barracuda, beluga, bluegill, clam, conch, crab, eel, flounder, frog, gray sole, haddock, halibut, pickled herring, lobster, lox, octopus, oysters, sea bass, shrimp, smoked salmon, striped bass, and turtle.

Some natural beans for group AB

Cat fish   tilapia fish   croaker fish

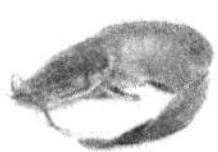 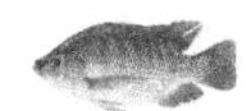 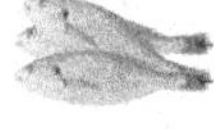

Some beneficial beans for group AB

Snail   sardine

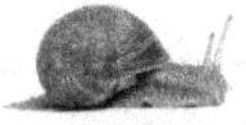 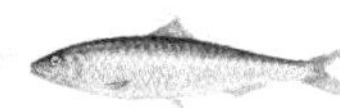

Salmon fish   red snapper fish

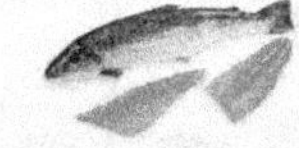 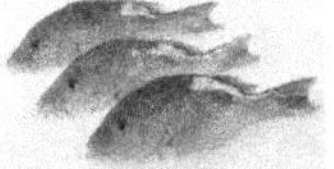

Some detrimental beans for group AB

Crab   octopi's fish

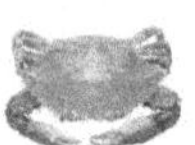 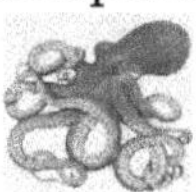

Barracuda fish crayfish

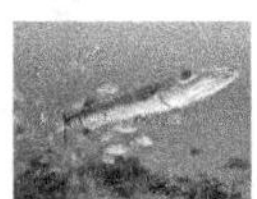 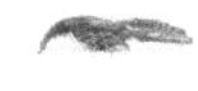

OILS AND FATS

Type AB's need very little fat to function well, but a tablespoon of **olive oil** on salads or steamed vegetables daily will aid digestion. Monounsaturated fatty acids (MUFAs) found in all kinds of olive oil are considered a healthy fat.

Some natural beans for group AB

Cod liver oil almond oil

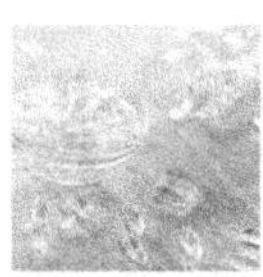 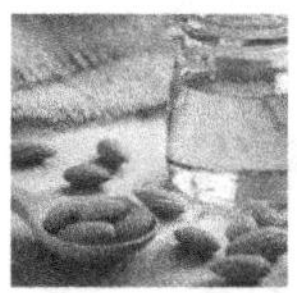

Some beneficial beans for group AB

Olive oil   walnut oil

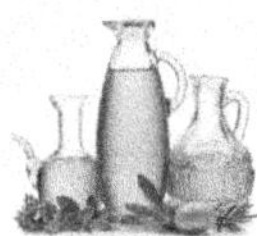 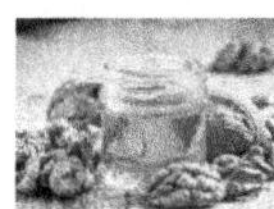

Some detrimental beans for group AB

Coconut oil   cotton seed oil

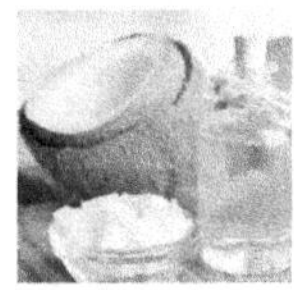 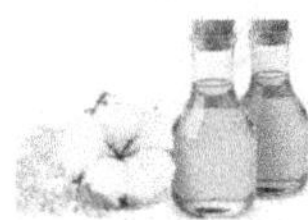

VEGETABLES

Fresh vegetables are an important source of Phyto-chemicals the natural substances in foods that have a tonic effect in cancer and heart disease prevention - diseases that afflict group A and group AB more often as a result of weaker immune systems. They should be eaten several times a day. Group AB have a wide selection- nearly all the vegetables that are good for either   Group A or B are good for you as well.

Some natural vegetables for group AB

Tomato   okra   carrot

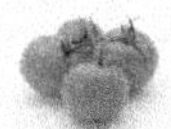 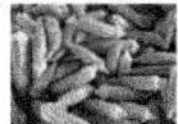 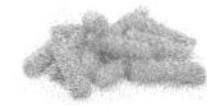

Ginger   pumpkin   onion

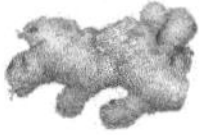 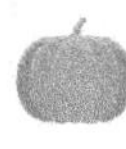 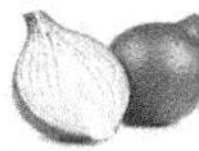

Spinach   lettuce   cabbage

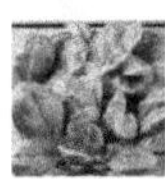 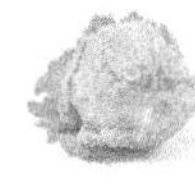 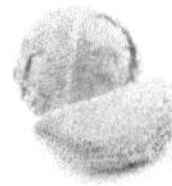

Some beneficial vegetables for group AB

Cucumber   garlic   mushroom

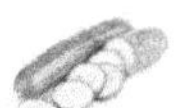 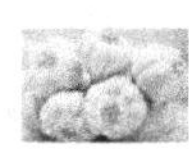 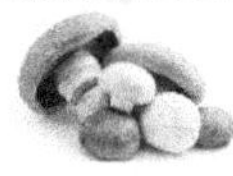

Sweet potato   eggplant   yam

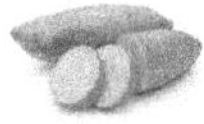 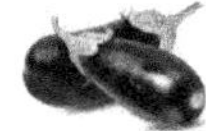 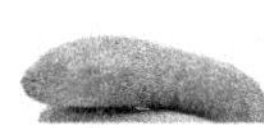

Some detrimental vegetables for group AB

Corn   aloe Vera   pepper

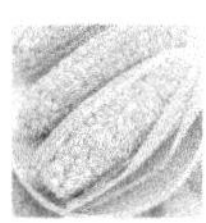 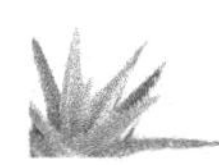 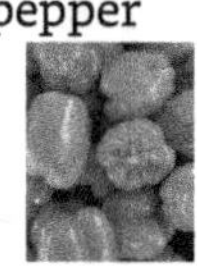

FRUIT

Group Abs inherit mostly group A in tolerance and preferences for certain fruits. Emphasize the more alkaline fruits, such as grapes, plums and berries, which can help to balance the grains that are acid forming in your muscle tissues. Group ABs don't do particularly well on certain tropical fruits in particular mangoes and guava. But pineapple is an excellent digestive aid for Group AB.

Some natural fruits for group AB

Apple   tangerine

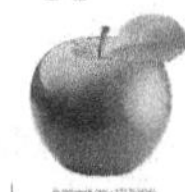 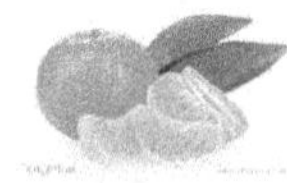

Pawpaw   melon

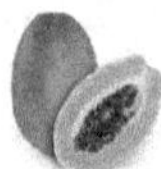 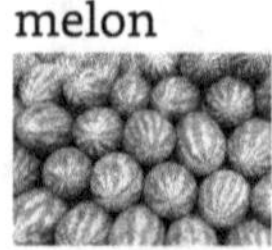

Some beneficial fruits for group AB

Pineapple   watermelon   lemon

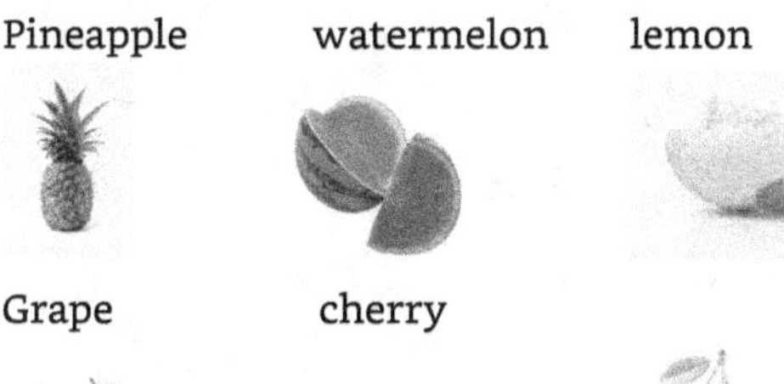

Grape   cherry

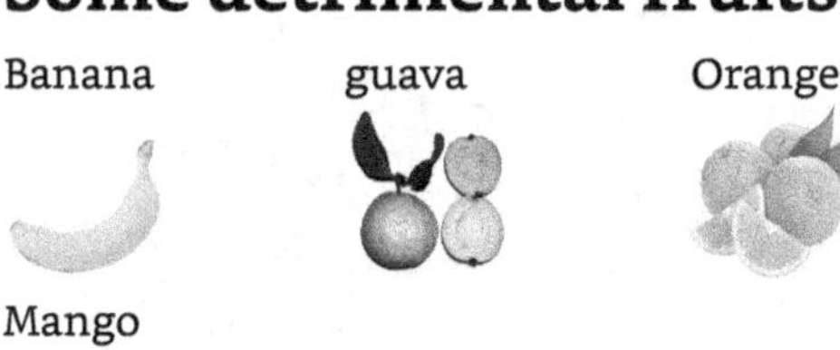

Some detrimental fruits for group AB

Banana   guava   Orange

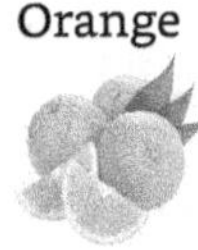

Mango

JUICES AND FLUIDS

Group AB should begin each da' by drinking a glass of warm Water with the freshly squeezed juice of half a lemon to cleanse the system of mucus accumulated while sleeping. The lemon water also aids elimination. Follow with a diluted glass of grapefruit or high alkaline fruit juices such as black cherry or grape.

Some natural juice for group AB

Grape juice   pineapple juice apple juice

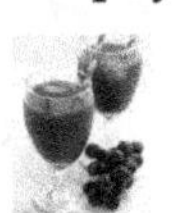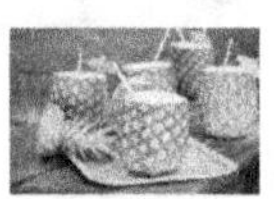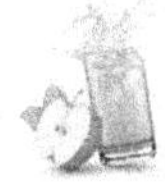

Cucumber juice pawpaw juice   tangerine juice

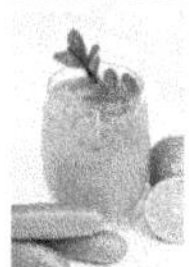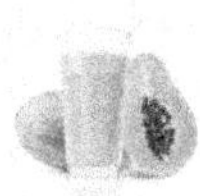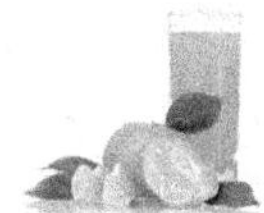

Some beneficial juice for group AB

Carrot juice   cherry juice

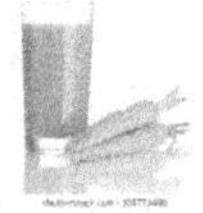 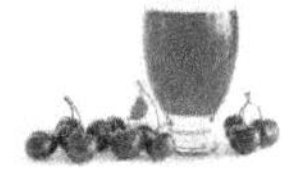

lemon juice   Cabbage juice

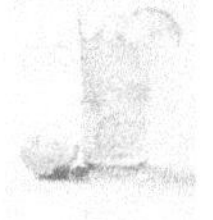 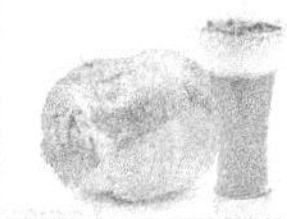

Some detrimental juice for group AB

Mango juice   guava juice   orange juice

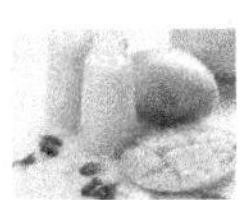 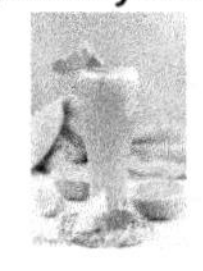 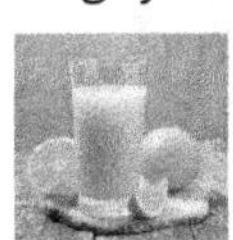

SPICES SUGARS AND SEASONINGS

Sea salt and kelp should be used in place of salt. Their sodium content is low-a concern for Group AB and kelp has immensely positive heart and immune system benefits. It is also useful for weight control. Miso, made from soy, is very good for Group AB, and makes a delicious soup or sauce. Avoid all pepper and vinegar because they are acidic.

Some natural spices, sugar and seasonings for group AB

Honey   salt   bay leaf

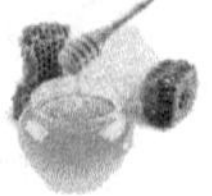 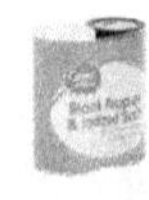 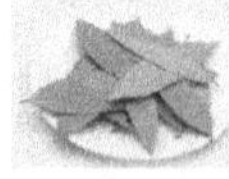

Sugar   nutmeg

 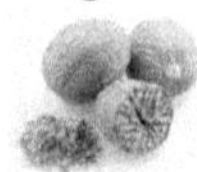

Some beneficial spices, sugar and seasonings for group AB

Curry   ginger   garlic

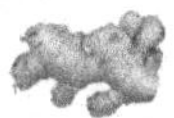 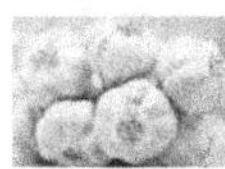

Some detrimental spices, sugar and seasonings for group AB

Corn syrup   vinegar

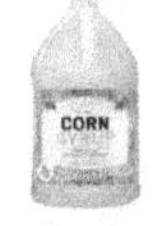 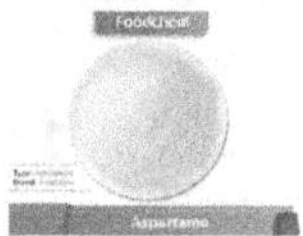

Aspartame   MSG

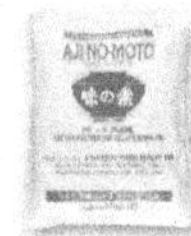

CONDIMENTS

Be sure to avoid all pickled condiments, due to a susceptibility stomach cancer. Also avoid ketchup which contains vinegar.

Some natural condiments for group AB

Mayonnaise apple butter jam jelly

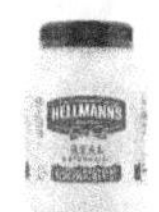 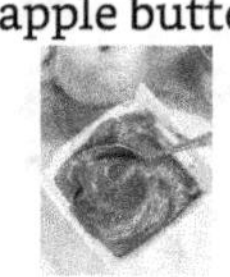 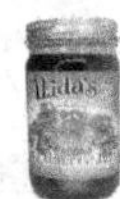

Some beneficial condiments for group AB

Oregano   blackstrap molasses

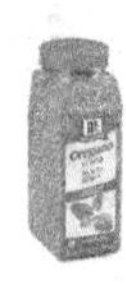 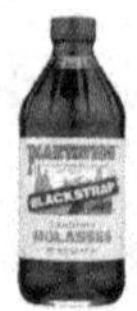

Some detrimental condiments for group AB

Pickle relish   ketchup   soy sauce

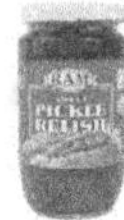 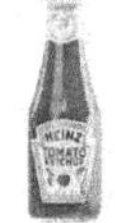 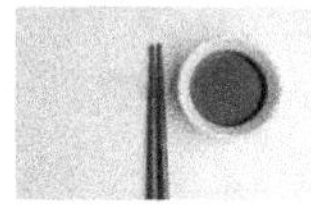

BEVERAGES

Red wine is good for Group AB because of its positive cardiovascular effects. A glass of red wine every day is believed to lower the risk of heart disease, for both men and women. Replace coffee with green tea for the greatest benefit.

Some natural beans for group AB

White wine   soda (club)

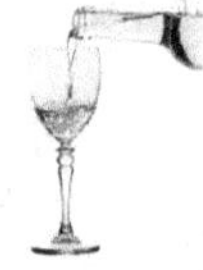 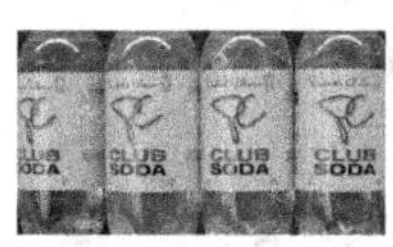

Red wine   seltzer water

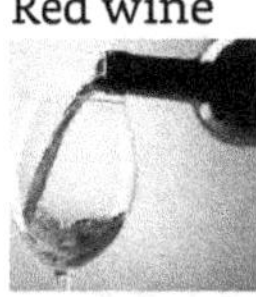 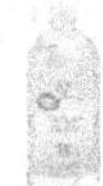

Some beneficial beans for group AB

Green teas

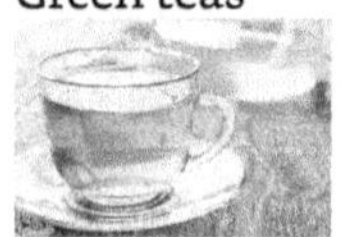

Some detrimental beans for group AB

Distilled   liquor

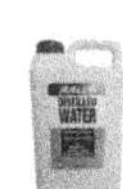 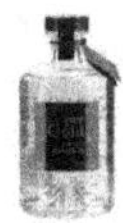

Black teas coffee (decaf/regular)

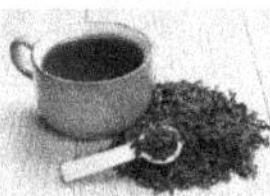 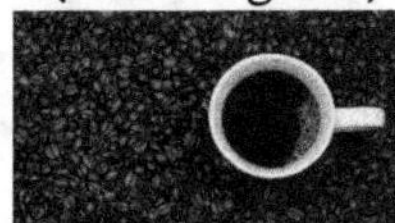

CHAPTER EIGTH

The right way to eat

Now that you have an understanding of what your food is, you also need to understand the right way of eating because it is not sufficient to eat the right food, there are right ways to eat to be healthy.

TEN RIGHT WAYS TO EAT

. 1. Eat the right food at the right time

Breakfast: (breakfast food is a food that is eaten primarily for the first meal of the day) 6am - 8a.m; Juices, Fluids or Cereals. If you must eat at early morning, let it be fluid, oatmeal, juices or cereals because your body is not equipped until late morning to digest heavy cooked carbohydrates.

Brunch: (Late Morning meal) 9a.m – 11a.m) Brunch is a late morning meal taken instead of breakfast and lunch. Brunch will replace breakfast and lunch. French toast, pancakes, Bread, Muffins, Grains or Pastas. Fruit: apples berries, melons and citrus fruits are popular side to have with brunch.

Lunch: (Mid-day meal12noon -2p.m: Cooked Vegetables include under root, bulb and leave vegetable. Eating lunch raises your blood sugar level in the middle of the day, which gives you the energy you need for the rest of the day. It also enables you to focus and concentrate on the rest of the afternoon.

Supper: it is related to the late afternoon or early evening meal. Supper is most often a light meal. 5p.m -7p.m: Raw vegetables, Fruits, Beans and Legumes, meat and poultry.

Avoid eating when you feel programed or stimulated hunger. Programmed hunger is when the body is programmed to eat food at a certain time, the bodies naturally and always ask for food at that particular time. For instance, let us assumed you are someone that eats supper 9p.m every time, your body will be programmed to ask for food at that time naturally. If by any chance you happen to eat supper by 7p.m one day you will observe that at the dot of 9p.m that day, you will feel hungry.

The hunger you feel at that time is programmed hunger. Stimulated hunger is when one body craves for food after one has perceived the aroma of food. You will observe that when you avoid eating when you feel programmed or stimulated hunger, after some time the craving will disappear.

2. Combine food properly A. Don't mix carbohydrate and protein heavy at the same time. Carbohydrate is digested in alkaline digestive juices while protein is digested in acid digestive juices. Eating food heavy in carbohydrate and protein at the same meal makes the alkaline and acid juices to neutralize each other, producing salt and water. This slows down digestion and leads to constipation.

B. Don't mix fast digesting and slow digesting fruits together. For instance, watermelon is very fast digesting. it takes about thirty to forty minutes to digest while banana is very slow to digest, it takes four hours to digest. When you take watermelon on banana, you are simply saying that watermelon should hold on for four hours for banana to digest first before it takes it turn and it doesn't work that way. In that case, watermelon will not digest, it will simply ferment.

C. Don't combine neutral foods together, take for instance, you are blood group O, you should not eat yam and egg together, they are both neutral in your system. You should rather eat sweet potato and egg together; your body will be better served. If you. Eat yarn; eat it with beef stew or sauce. That's combining neutral with beneficial.

3. Eat slowly

When you eat slowly, you give time for your brain to signal to your stomach that you are full, this way, you will guide against over-eating.

4. Masticate or chew food properly

You need to chew your food properly because digestion of food starts from mouth as you mix plenty of saliva with your food.

5. Don't drink water while eating Drinking water while eating will dilute your digestive juices and slow down digestion.

6. Stay without food sometimes

You need to stay without food for once m a week or at least thrice m a month this will allow your digestive system to go on break and rest

7. Don't eat under stress or distress Digestion is impaired when you eat under stress, distress or anxiety. 8. Don't eat while watching television or while working on computer, you need to concentrate on your meal while eating Avoid distraction

9. Eat a balanced diet A balanced diet should include raw and cooked foods. For, instance cooked rice should be eaten alongside some raw vegetables or fruits

10. Don't overeat

Don't eat to the point that you start to feel dizzy When you do, you have forced some of your organs to switch off, especially your brain. They were forced to switch off to give room for your digestive system to have enough power to digest your food. This explains the dizziness Also try to eat based on the level of your activity. If you are a banker don't eat like a mechanic. Learn to count calories. Your daily need of calories is a function of your level of activity. The table below shows the different calories need of different level of activity.

Types of Activity	Profession	Daily Calories Intake
Very Light	Teachers. Bankers	1 800

Light	Students. Sales men	2 300
Moderate	Mechanics. Carpenters	2 800
Intense	Athletes. Miners	3 500

You must balance your intake of calories from food with the energy you use in everyday activities.

The two forms of healthy food preparation that I will like to recommend are baking and boiling. Bake and boil your food. Avoid roasting and frying.

Baking is a method of cooking food that uses prolonged dry heat normally in an oven but also in hot ashes or on hot stone while boiling is the method of cooking food in bailing water or water like substances.

Frying on the other hand is the cooking of food in fat. This takes several forms, from deep frying where the food is completely immersed in hot oil or where food is cooked in a frying pan where there is only a thin coating of oil. Frying is unhealthy because if you fry your food in a type of fat that produces a lot Is of saturated fat, it may increase your cholesterol and your risk of heart disease, Roasting is a cooking method that uses dry heat where hot air envelops the food, cooking it evenly on all sides from an open flame oven or other heat source. When you roast food until it gets dark and crispy, it releases harmful free radicals.

Food Preparation Tools

There are basic tools that are necessary for healthy food preparations:

1. **Blender:** it has many uses in the kitchen from blending pepper to making smoothies and so much more. Avoid the use of commercial grinding machine; inexpensive blender from a discount office will do a reasonable job. S

2. **Oven and cooking gas**: an oven and a cooking gas will make your food preparation easier, faster and healthier. They come in various sizes and prizes.

3. **Refrigerator:** this is needed for food preservation, lf you need to preserve food, use refrigerator. You have no need of freezer. Frozen

foods are unhealthy the fresher your food the healthier it is.

4. **Pots and Pans:** Aluminum pots and pans are perfectly safe, about half of all cookware is aluminum. Pots and pans made from aluminum and stainless steel have nearly replaced the cast iron pots of old but they are no match for them. The biggest practical difference is nothing sticks to a well-seasoned cast iron pan, while everything sticks to cast aluminum.

Healthy Food Preparation Tips

1. Go an extra mile to organize your food items: To get natural and organic foods. You need to go far.

2. Spend quality time in your food preparation: Avoid instant preparation of foods. Take time to add beneficial ingredients.

3. Always make health a priority in your food preparation: Think of health first before taste and aroma.

CHAPTER NINE

Adaptation of Normal Diet for Changing Needs

Normal Diet

Normal Diet is modified to take care of small kids, old individuals and debilitated individuals from the family. The preparation of diet whether typical, soft or liquid has a similar fundamental goal — to keep up with, or reestablish the great strength of the individual through a proper diet. The modifications depend on the changed requirements of the individual, due to age or sickness.

Normal Diet shapes the premise of all modifications of diets for age and ailment; yet due consideration should be paid to needs of the individual. Normal diet is arranged by the recommended everyday dietary admissions, which are intended to address the issues of every healthy person and may not address the issues of sick persons. The nutritional requirements rely upon the activity, the expanded or diminished requests for specific supplements, which should be viewed as in planning the diet.

The arrangement given in Table 23.1 for a typical eating routine might be adjusted to suit different social or financial conditions. Alterations of Normal Diet: The ordinary eating regimen might be changed to1. Provide change in consistency, e.g., soft and fluid diets;

2. Provide foods bland in flavor;

3. Modify intervals of feeding;

4. Increase or decrease energy content;

5. Increase or decrease other nutrients, e.g., protein;

6. Increase or decrease fibred.

Liquid and Soft Diets

The kind of modification connects with the condition and need of the individual concerned. The choice of food sources is made on similar standards as the normal diet, using the daily food guide.

Mechanical Soft Diet: Many individuals, including newborn children, need soft diet since they have no teeth. Hence, the main change made is in the consistency of the food sources served. No limitation is put on food selection. This diet is sometimes described as mechanically soft diet

Table: Normal Diet

Food Group	Foods to be Included	Amount
1	Rice Chapati/Roti Upma/Shira/Poche Bread. etc.	6 or more servings
2.	Milk	2-3 Servings
	Dal	2 or more servings
	Egg/Fish/Meat, if acceptable	2 or more servings
3(a)	Leafy vegetables	1 or more servings
3(b)	Citrus or other vitamin-C rich fruits	1 or more servings
4.	Other vegetables, fruits and Roots, tubers	2 or more servings
5.	Oil	15 g or more as required

Sugar/Butter/Ghee/Vanaspati   to meet energy needs

The following changes in the normal diet will meet the needs of individuals without teeth:

• Rice and other cereals to be served soft-cooked.

• Chapati/roti/bread—soft breads are substituted for hard, crusty preparations.

• Dal and whole pulses must be cooked thoroughly.

• Eggs—boiled or scrambled. •

Meat/fish should be ground or minced finely. •

Cooked vegetables may be used.

 Most raw vegetables are omitted, except tomatoes, finely chopped cucumber, lettuce, coriander, and mint (pudina). Chutney may be acceptable.

• Raw fruits, which are juicy and soft can be included—banana, mango (non-fibrous varieties), oranges, musambi, grape fruit, soft berries, jack fruit (soft variety), all melons, grapes, with soft skins, soft pear, peaches, apricots, plums (minus skins), etc.

• Apples may be served after cooking or baking.

• Tough skins, stones, fibers should be removed from fruits and vegetables, e.g., apple skin, potato skin, etc.

• Nuts and dried fruits need to be finely ground, when used. Soft Diet: It is a step between the full liquid and the normal diet. It is served to persons suffering from acute infections, gastrointestinal disturbances or persons recovering from surgery. The diet consists of simple soft foods, which are easy to chew and easy to digest. Harsh fibred, fatty or highly spiced foods are avoided. It is nutritionally adequate, when planned according to the Daily Food Guide. The soft diet includes:

• Soft cooked rice, soft chapati and bread—6 servings or more

• Milk, dahl (curd), buttermilk, paneer, soft cheese—2-3 servings

• Dals, well-cooked—2-3 servings

• Eggs poached, boiled, trader ground meat, fish and poultry—2-3 servings

• Vegetables and fruits made up of 1. Green leafy vegetables cooked and strained—2-3 servings 2. Citrus fruits or juice or mango (non-

fibrous varieties)—2-3 servings
 • Other vegetables and fruits, not mentioned above, such as:
1. other vegetables—tender, chopped and cooked—2-3 servings
2. Other fruits—banana or cooked fruits without skin or seeds—2-3 servings.
Additional foods such as butter, soups, soft desserts (such as kheer/payasam) and more of the above foods can be included to meet the nutritional needs. The following foods are avoided:
• Legumes (whole).
• Egg (fried).
• Meat, tough, salted, smoked fish or meat.
• Vegetables and fruits raw, except those mentioned above; strongly flavored ones.
• Bread and cereals coarse, with bran, whole-grain preparations and fatty recipes.
• Soups—fatty or highly seasoned.
• Fats—fried foods, e.g., potato chips.
• Miscellaneous: hot flavors, pickles, nuts, and so forth. Liquid Diets or full liquid weight control plans are ready for people experiencing fevers, people who have recently gone through operation or whenever a person is unable to tolerate solid foods. The adequacy of such a diet will rely upon the kinds of liquids permitted.
Full liquid diet is served to people, who are extremely sick and can't bite or swallow strong food. It incorporates all food varieties, which are liquid at 37°C. To keep away from difficulty in swallowing, fibrous food varieties and irritating flavors are excluded from this diet. The time of use of this diet relies upon the state of the patient. As the supplement content is diluted, the interval between feeds is reduced and the number of feeds is increased to six or more.
The protein content of the eating regimen can be expanded by adding skimmed milk powder in the soups and refreshments. Cooked, crushed dal can be utilized to get ready soups. Stressed, ground meat or fish can be added to stocks.
The energy content of the diet can be increased by adding

expanded by adding (a) cream to drain, (b) margarine/oil to oat slops and dal soups, (c) glucose to juices, milk, (d) involving cream in pastries.

The following foods can be included in the full fluid diet:
• Milk—1 liter
• Eggs—2 (in custard or in eggnog)
• Dal, well-cooked—25–50 g
• Meat/fish cooked and strained—25-50 g
• Cereal strained—1/2 cup (100 g) cooked as gruel
• Vegetables—1/4 cup cooked, strained or puree for soup
• Fruit juices—1 cup, citrus and other strained juices
• Tomato or vegetable juices—1/2 cup
• Butter
• Sugar
• Kheer, ice-cream, gelatin dessert, custard
• Soups—broth
• Tea, coffee, soft drinks
• Flavorings, salt. Clear liquid diet is given when an individual can't endure food, because of sickness, heaving, gas formation, diarrhea, or outrageous absence of appetite. This diet is allowed for a little while, until the patient can take a more liberal fluid diet. As the name shows the diet comprises of clear fluids like tea with lemon and sugar, coffee, grain removes (extract of puffed cereals also), strained organic product juices, carbonated drinks, dal extract, fat-free stock, and so on. The sum is confined to 30 to 60 ml each hour first and foremost and continuously expanded. This diet replaces the liquids lost by the body, thus preventing dehydration.

Ongoing pattern is to assist the patient with advancing from clear liquid to liquid too soft to mechanically soft to normal diet as quickly as possible. Consequently, the deficiency of the primary phase of diet may not influence the patient's wellbeing unfavorably, as he is urged to get through this stage in a day or two.

www.ingramcontent.com/pod-product-compliance
Lightning Source LLC
Chambersburg PA
CBHW050039260726
48658CB00005B/1678